LATER

Roger H. S. Carpenter was formerly Professor of Oculomotor Physiology, University of Cambridge and Tutor, Registrary and Director of Studies in Medicine, Gonville & Caius College. He was the creator of EPIC (the Experimental Physiology Instrumentation Computer) and NeuroLab, a set of interactive demonstrations on the working of the human brain. He was an influential scientist and passionate teacher of neurophysiology, collaborating with Dr Noorani on the project before his death in 2019. Professor Carpenter made lasting contributions to the field of neurophysiology and is widely regarded as an exceptional mentor by a plethora of his former students.

Imran Noorani is a Neurosurgery NIHR Clinical Lecturer at University College London (Institute of Neurology). He worked closely with Professor Carpenter to advance the LATER model to more complex decision processes in the laboratory, such as antisaccades. Dr Noorani has won multiple awards for his research, including the European Association of Neurosurgical Societies Award for Best Laboratory Research 2020, and in addition to clinical and research interests, has a strong interest in teaching undergraduates.

"Why are reaction times so long and so variable? Synthesizing a lifetime's work, *LATER* both quantitatively and philosophically describes why our brains deliberately exploit procrastination and randomness. Carpenter's dual role as neuroscientist and teacher is on full display here, with potentially tricky principles and concepts explained with exceptional clarity. An essential reference for anyone with an interest in response times and decision-making."

Andrew Anderson
The University of Melbourne

"Overall, simplicity in explanations promotes effective communication, enhances understanding, and ensures that information is accessible to a broader audience. The *LATER* model introduced by Roger Carpenter is "simple." Notably, a simple model gives trackable hypotheses and testable predictions for neurophysiological processes responsible for behavior. I am tremendously missing the discussions with Roger Carpenter. I'll never forget my first visit to Cambridge and our discussion in the smoking salon. I was a young scientist, and Roger Carpenter was an established Professor; exchanging without any barrier on freewill, variability, and "noise," as well as poetry, was very revealing to me and is still a source of inspiration. I rarely encounter such personal attention during my career. I trust that some aspects of these discussions will remain perennial throughout this book. I'm convinced some of these ideas will be passed to more generations of students and young or less young researchers in multiple interdisciplinary fields in neurosciences."

Pierre Pouget
Director of Research at CNRS (Brain Institute) Paris

LATER

The Neurophysiology of Decision-Making

Roger H. S. Carpenter
Late of Gonville and Caius College, Cambridge

Imran Noorani
University College London

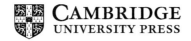

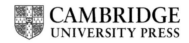

Shaftesbury Road, Cambridge CB2 8EA, United Kingdom

One Liberty Plaza, 20th Floor, New York, NY 10006, USA

477 Williamstown Road, Port Melbourne, VIC 3207, Australia

314–321, 3rd Floor, Plot 3, Splendor Forum, Jasola District Centre, New Delhi – 110025, India

103 Penang Road, #05-06/07, Visioncrest Commercial, Singapore 238467

Cambridge University Press is part of Cambridge University Press & Assessment, a department of the University of Cambridge.

We share the University's mission to contribute to society through the pursuit of education, learning and research at the highest international levels of excellence.

www.cambridge.org
Information on this title: www.cambridge.org/9781108827041

DOI: 10.1017/9781108920803

First published 2023

Printed in the United Kingdom by CPI Group Ltd, Croydon CR0 4YY

A catalogue record for this publication is available from the British Library.

Library of Congress Cataloging-in-Publication Data
Names: Carpenter, R. H. S. (Roger H. S.), 1945-2017, author. |
    Noorani, Imran, author.
Title: LATER : the neurophysiology of decision-making /
    Roger H. S. Carpenter, Imran Noorani.
Other titles: Neurophysiology of decision-making
Description: Cambridge, United Kingdom ; New York, NY :
    Cambridge University Press, 2023. | Includes bibliographical references and index.
Identifiers: LCCN 2023004594 (print) | LCCN 2023004595 (ebook) |
    ISBN 9781108827041 (paperback) | ISBN 9781108920803 (epub)
Subjects: MESH: Decision Making–physiology | Procrastination–
    physiology | Linear Models | Models, Neurological
Classification: LCC BF448 (print) | LCC BF448 (ebook) |
    NLM BF 448 | DDC 153.8/3–dc23/eng/20230309
LC record available at https://lccn.loc.gov/2023004594
LC ebook record available at https://lccn.loc.gov/2023004595

ISBN 978-1-108-82704-1 Paperback

....

Contents

Preface

Science progresses by flashes of ignorance, when we suddenly realise we don't actually understand some phenomenon we have long taken for granted. A particularly striking example is *Why is deciding to do something so slow?* Nerves and muscles are not to blame; rather, it is an example of *procrastination*: the higher areas of the brain deliberately suppress lower areas capable of generating much faster but ill-considered responses while they elaborate more sophisticated ones. So, reaction time is decision time, and it can tell us a great deal about how decisions are made – the very highest level of cerebral function, the most difficult faced by the brain. It is also ultimately the scariest – a matter of life and death. We have to decide whether the investment of energy in making a particular response is likely to be greater or less than what is gained in return. In this book we trace the development of these ideas, focusing especially on a particular model, LATER, that despite being very simple, explains these decision mechanisms in quantitative detail.

Acknowledgements

This little book has been very long in gestation (over ten years), but with a remarkably rapid birth (those who enjoy irony will see that this is all too reminiscent of the LATER model itself). The reason for the slow rise to threshold was a diagnosis of a terminal illness, so my first thanks need to be to those who have provided the remarkable clinical care that I have received at Addenbrooke's Hospital. It is invidious to single out individuals from a universally excellent team, but particular thanks must go to Dr Charles Crawley and Dr Kumar Kumararatne for keeping me alive during this period.

I could not have done this without the love and support of my wife, Christine, on whom the immense burden of day-to-day care during my illness has fallen. I am more grateful to her than I can express. And also my children, Jamie and Alison, for their ongoing support an encouragement during a difficult period.

Finally, Dr Imran Noorani, also of Addenbrooke's Hospital previously, has very kindly taken on oversight of final publication of this book.

Roger H. S. Carpenter

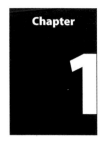

The Slowness of Reaction Time

They are ill discoverers that think there is no land, when they can see nothing but sea.
Francis Bacon, The Advancement of Learning *(1605)*

There are two kinds of science.

Usually it is a matter of systematic and patient collection of data, testing hypotheses that consolidate our knowledge in the vicinity of what we already know. We record the effect of altering this or that experimental condition, and gradually the area of scientific terra firma encroaches on the ocean of ignorance: slowly but surely the shoreline extends, creating the branched causeway we regard as Truth.

But a riskier approach is to look farther out to sea: to have hunches about what direction the advance is going to take and carry out speculative experiments. Often they fail: but if they work, by indicating the direction that needs to be taken, they can speed things up enormously.

Interpolation and extrapolation: and on the whole – possibly unfairly – it is the extrapolators who get remembered as the scientific giants. The training of scientists tends to focus on the first kind of science, on the systematic design of experiments, the unbiased assessment of statistical results, thorough assimilation of the literature, ensuring that one's own little pebble is firmly bedded and securely attached to its neighbours. Rather little is ever said about how to encourage the process that generates sudden leaps of the scientific imagination. The problem is partly that knowledge inhibits imagination; it takes a great deal of intellectual effort to look at phenomena with an innocent eye. The story of Newton and the falling apple is meant to illustrate this. Falling is so universal a phenomenon that we take it for granted; what Newton realised was that the acceleration implied that gravity was some kind of force that attracted the moon in the same way as the apple. As Isaac Asimov has put it (Asimov 1984), 'The most exciting phrase to hear in science, the one that heralds new discoveries, is not Eureka! but That's funny!'

This book is about trying to explain just such a phenomenon: one that we experience in ourselves every moment of our lives, that until a few decades ago had never been recognised for the mystery that it evidently is. That phenomenon is *reaction time*, the delay or latency between stimulus and response. Why do we take so long to respond to things? The attempt to answer that question turns out to shed light on some of the most fundamental processes within the brain, processes that lie right at the top of the brain's organisational hierarchy and are linked in a profound way with some of the deepest mysteries of cerebral function – consciousness, creativity, free will.

Although there are many kinds of stimuli to which we respond, with many kinds of responses, certain features of reaction times seem to be remarkably constant. The best-studied example is a movement we take for granted, though we do it more often than any other – two or three times every second of our waking life – far commoner, for instance, than the heartbeat. Since it forms the focus of much of this book, it may be helpful at this point to have a brief digression to introduce it. It is a common eye movement called a saccade, whose function is to move our gaze from one object to another. Because we make so many of them, with modern equipment that measures saccades non-invasively and automatically, we can record thousands of saccades in an afternoon and obtain very precise information about their latencies.

1.1 Saccades

To be short, they be wholly given to follow the motions of the minde, they doe change themselves in a moment, they doe alter and conforme themselves unto it in such manner, as that Blemor the Arabian, and Syerneus the Phisition of Cypres, thought it no absurditie to affirme that the soule dwelt in the eyes . . .
A. Laurentius (A du Laurens), A Discourse of the Preservation of Sight *(1599)*

Eye movements evolved in order to make up for various deficiencies in our vision (Helmholtz 1867, Carpenter 1992a, Land 1995, Land and Tatler 2009). The most fundamental is that retinal receptors are slow to respond to visual stimuli. As a result, they cannot cope with an image that is moving, and therefore generating retinal slip. The first eye movements to evolve were *gaze-holding* movements, designed to eliminate retinal slip by using visual feedback (optokinetic responses), and predictive information about head movement from the vestibular system. Gaze is not the same as eye position: it means the direction of the line of sight relative to the outside world, whereas eye position means the direction of the line of sight relative to the head. Gaze is *craniocentric* and determines where images of objects fall on the retina; eye position is *retinocentric*; to convert one into the other, we need to know our head position (Carpenter 1988).

The second defect is that the retina of the eye is not uniformly excellent. Right in the middle is an area where the cone receptors are tightly packed and the overlying layers of neurons are pushed to one side, producing the very best possible visual acuity. But elsewhere the rod receptors – specialised for vision at night – are mingled with cones, and the optics are not optimal. Furthermore, the signals from the retinal receptors tend to be pooled before entering the optic nerve. This convergence is necessary if the optic nerve is to be of a manageable size: although we have some 120 million receptors in each eye, the number of fibres in the optic nerve is only a million or so. The consequence of all this is that although when we enter a new set of surroundings, we have the illusion that we can see everything equally clearly; this is not the case. Only a very small area immediately around our point of gaze, the fovea, enjoys detailed vision: as we go farther out, things are increasingly blurred (Figure 1.1).

The illusion of universal clear vision comes about because the eye jumps rapidly from one place to another within the scene, getting information about detail that is then stored and forms the basis of our perception (Figure 1.1). These jumps are called *saccades* (from a French word meaning 'jerks') and are examples of gaze-shifting movements. As William Porterfield wrote in 1737 (Porterfield 1737), '. . . *in viewing any large Body, we are ready to imagine we see at the same Time all its Parts equally distinct and clear: But*

(a)   (b)   (c)

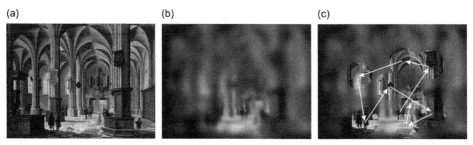

Figure 1.1 (a) On entering an unfamiliar space, we seem to see it all at once. But this is an illusion, for we know that only the central foveal region actually transmits information to the brain with sufficient acuity; what actually happens is that we rapidly scan the area with a series of saccades (b), piecing together this foveal information into a seamless whole (c). (Interior of the Cunerakerk, Rhenen (1638): National Gallery, London.)

(a)   (b)

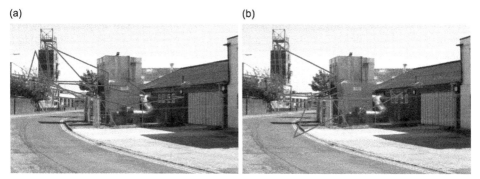

Figure 1.2 Saccadic trajectories (in red, a,b) made by two different subjects viewing the same scene on a computer monitor (courtesy of Dr Benjamin Tatler).

this is a vulgar Error, and we are led into it from the quick and almost continual Motion of the Eye, whereby it is successively directed towards all the Parts of the Object in an Instant of Time.' Figure 1.2 shows sequences of saccades made by two different subjects viewing a detailed scene suddenly presented to them. You can see that there is a tendency for the saccades to concentrate on the more interesting parts of the scene, those most likely to provide information and requiring detailed visual analysis: blank areas such as sky are on the whole left alone.

A great deal can be learned from spontaneous saccades of this kind, in particular about the mechanisms that determine what is most likely to be chosen as a target. But as so often in behavioural science, there is a kind of tension between the desire to investigate situations that are 'ecological' – as natural and realistic as possible, with the minimum of instructions to the subject as to what they are supposed to do – and the benefits of a controlled laboratory environment with highly constrained tasks and simple, abstract targets. The former are more 'real', but generate messy data; the latter can produce precise quantitative results that lend themselves to exact modelling. But they tell us only about a very artificial situation.

The findings that form the subject of this book have come almost entirely from experiments of the second kind, from evoked saccades rather than from spontaneous ones; though they are applicable to more natural situations as well, as we shall see in Section 4.8.

1.1.1 The Step Task

The simplest of all these evoked tasks is the *step task*. A subject is presented with a small, central visual target and asked to look at it and follow it with their gaze if it moves. A single trial might begin with the target presented centrally, and then – after a delay – jumping either to the left or to the right (Figure 1.3). Both the direction and the delay need to be randomised on each trial, because – as we shall see in Section 3.4 – the saccadic system is extremely intelligent, quickly adapting its behaviour in response to any aspect of the protocol that is predictable (Figure 1.4).

Figure 1.5 shows the outcome of one such trial. In response to the step movement of the target, the eye moves precisely and extremely rapidly from its initial central location to its new position, in this case a movement of 5 degrees (deg). Saccades such as these are some of the fastest movements the body makes: in this case, the movement is over in about 30 milliseconds (ms), and the peak velocity of the eye in large saccades can be many hundreds of degrees per second. These speeds have evolved because the visual system is effectively blind during a saccade, so the shorter they last, the better (Dodge 1900, 1905).

But this record also demonstrates something very strange indeed. A saccade is a masterpiece of biological engineering, throwing the gaze neatly on to a visual target by a

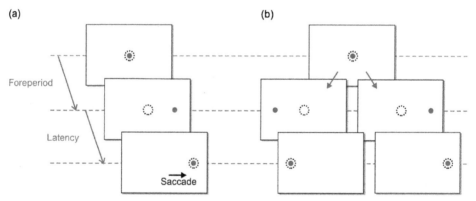

Figure 1.3 A saccadic protocol: the step task. (a) The target (red) is fixated (the dotted circle shows eye position); then after a foreperiod of random duration, it jumps to one side, followed by a saccade as the eye tracks it. The time between target and eye movement is the reaction time or latency. (b) A fully balanced task: after the foreperiod, the target may jump to left or right, at random.

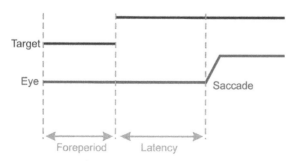

Figure 1.4 The timing of events in a typical step trial. After the foreperiod, the target jumps to one side; then after the reaction time or latency, the eye makes a saccade to the target. The experimenter will normally arrange for the foreperiod to vary randomly from trial to trial, as well as the direction of the target jump.

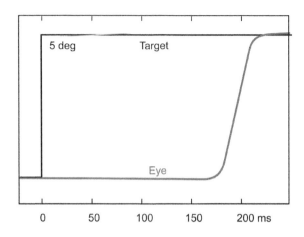

Figure 1.5 A saccade (red) in response to a 5-deg step of a visual target. Although the saccade itself only lasts an impressively short 30 ms, there is a latency of over 170 ms before the eye starts to move at all.

carefully programmed pattern of acceleration and deceleration that can last as little as 20–30 ms, at speeds of up to 800 deg/second (s) (Dodge and Cline 1901). Yet in another sense, saccades are surprisingly slow: saccadic latency is almost an order of magnitude longer than this, at around 200 ms.

An analogy may make it clearer just how bizarre this is. A fire station receives an urgent message: the Town Hall is on fire! Yet for an hour nothing seems to happen. Then suddenly the fire station doors are flung open, an engine emerges at top speed and arrives at the fire within a minute.

Why does it take nearly 200 ms after the target has been presented for the eye to start to move at all? Why has the evolutionary pressure to make the duration short not been matched by equal pressure to reduce the extreme slowness of the reaction time? This paradox is what this book is all about.

1.2 Procrastination

One of the lines of experimental investigation most diligently followed of late years is that of the ascertainment of the time occupied by nervous events. Helmholtz led off by discovering the rapidity of the current in the sciatic nerve of the frog. But the methods he used were soon applied to the sensory nerves and the centres, and the results caused much popular scientific admiration when described as measurements of the 'velocity of thought'.
William James, Principles of Psychology *(1890)*

Of course, many physical and physiological processes have to happen, one after another, to allow the eye to move to a visual stimulus. Are these components long enough to explain those 200 ms? A physiologist would immediately think of all the neural events that necessarily cause delay between a stimulus and a response. Every synapse between one neuron and the next introduces a small delay, as do the visual receptors of the eye, and the muscle fibres that eventually move it. And we also need to think about how fast the nerve fibres themselves are. We are used to wires that carry messages at around the speed of light, and computers whose rapidity is measured in nanoseconds; but even in the very fastest nerves the impulses or action potentials that carry information travel at a modest 100 m/s.

On the other hand, the distances are short: in this case, the most direct route linking the optic nerve to the eye muscles goes through a structure at the back of the brainstem

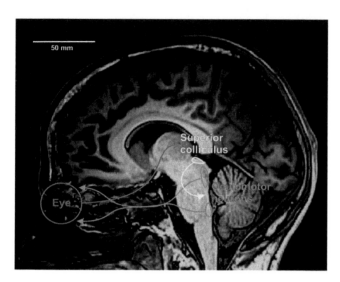

Figure 1.6 Midline section of human brain, showing the position of the superior colliculus in relation to the eye, and the oculomotor neurons in the brainstem that drive the eye muscles.
(Adapted from Wikimedia Commons under license from Creative Commons.)

called the superior colliculus (Crosby and Henderson 1948), and cannot be much more than some 10 centimetres (cm) (Figure 1.6). So even at 10 meters (m)/s this conduction time can't be more than 10 ms. Then there is the synaptic delay of 1 ms or so every time information passes from one neuron to the next; the collicular route involves perhaps 10 synapses at most, from retinal receptor to muscle fibre, adding a further 10 ms. The retinal receptors are themselves quite slow to respond to light, so this might account for perhaps 30 ms; and we need to add on perhaps 10 ms for muscle activation and tension development. In all, then, perhaps 60 ms: not negligible, but only about a third of the delay actually observed. In fact, it is not difficult to confirm these estimates directly. If we stimulate the colliculus of a monkey electrically, realistic saccades are produced, with a delay of about 20 ms (Robinson 1972); it is also possible to record collicular responses to visual stimulation, for which the delay is about 40 ms (Wurtz and Albano 1980). So our rather crude estimate turns out to be about right.

So why are saccadic latencies very much longer than simple considerations of conduction and transduction times would lead us to expect? The fundamental reason is that the colliculus is not very intelligent. It is both a sensory and motor structure: recording electrical responses evoked by small stimuli at different visual locations reveals that it maintains a systematic map of the visual world (Cynader and Berman 1972). Conversely, electrical stimulation at different locations on the superior collicular surface evokes saccades directed in a systematic way to corresponding points on this map (Robinson 1972). So here is an efficient neural device that translates the positions of visual targets into saccades that land on them: exactly what is needed to generate eye movements to look at objects presented at different locations. If the world consisted of single, localised targets in a darkened room, it would function beautifully. But it would be unable to cope even with two stimuli, let alone the huge number of interesting objects out there in the real visual world at any moment.

Worse, it lacks the kind of information it would need to decide which stimuli are actually worth looking at. The function of the superior collicular visual cells is limited essentially to determining *where* a target is: they have no idea *what* they are. Left to itself,

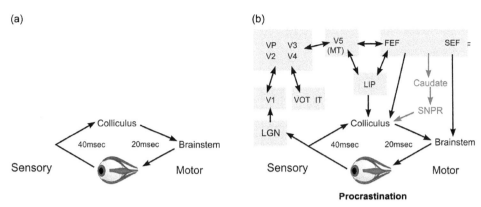

Figure 1.7 Highly schematic diagrams of direct and indirect pathways by which visual information could trigger a saccade. (a) The simple direct route through the colliculus that carries information about location but not much else. (b) Ascending pathways involving the lateral geniculate nucleus and a variety of cortical areas estimate whether a target is worth looking at. There is tonic descending inhibition, partly via structures in the basal ganglia that normally prevent the colliculus from making fast but erroneous saccades, which is then lifted locally to allow the colliculus to make a more thoughtfully directed saccade. LGN, lateral geniculate; V1, V2, V3, V4, V5, visual cortical areas; LIP, lateral inferior parietal area; FEF, frontal eye field; SEF, supplementary eye field; VP, ventral posterior area; MT, middle temporal area; VOT, ventral occipitotemporal cortex; IT, inferior temporal cortex.

and in conjunction with other subcortical areas such as the cerebellum, it has all the neural machinery needed to detect the position of a visual object and trigger an appropriately directed movement from the brainstem. But the real world is full of objects, some nice, some nasty, some familiar and safe, some demanding our immediate attention. The superior colliculus is incapable of choosing between them for the very good reason that its neurons have no idea what they are looking at: they respond directly neither to form nor to colour: clearly, they cannot be allowed to determine what we see. This requires much more complex analysis, to which the cerebral cortex in particular seems to be well suited. This kind of processing is more time-consuming than simple mapping. So while these more sophisticated judgements are being made, these higher, cortical, levels must tonically suppress the colliculus, preventing it from making over-fast, simple-minded responses (Figure 1.7).

Figure 1.7(a) shows this older and simpler visual pathway through the colliculus. But a huge amount of visual information takes a quite different route. Via a thalamic nucleus, the lateral geniculate (LGN), this information projects to visual cortical area V1 (striate cortex), and thence, directly or indirectly, to many other cortical areas responsible for analysing the attributes – colour, form and motion – of the retinal image (Figure 1.7(b)). These in turn project both to areas that are not wholly visual, such as the lateral inferior parietal area (LIP), and to areas that are specifically oculomotor, the frontal and supplementary eye fields (FEF and SEF). So there are many routes by which all these areas influence the superior colliculus and the areas of the brainstem concerned with controlling saccades. Many of them are tonically inhibitory, that is, their default is to inhibit saccade initiation. Corresponding to this continuing suppression, there are many inhibitory pathways that descend from cortex, such as the basal ganglia, that fire continuously, often at a very high rate, until the cortex has finished working out what movement to make next. This blanket of inhibition is lifted in a single localised area

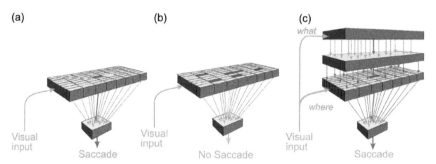

Figure 1.8 (a) The superior colliculus copes well if there is only one target, but not if there are many of them (b). Descending tonic inhibition is then needed (c), which is locally lifted when the decision has been made.

(Figure 1.8(a)), permitting the superior colliculus to carry out its basic function of converting visual location into an appropriately directed eye movement (Hikosaka and Wurtz 1983a, 1983b, 1983c, 1983d, Wurtz and Goldberg 1989, Hikosaka, Takikawa et al. 2000). In a sense, they can be thought of as preventing the collicular route from operating, so that reaction times are longer than they might otherwise be.

In other words, latency is mainly due not to conduction along nerves and across synapses, or the time taken to activate receptors and muscles (as is obvious from a second mysterious property mentioned earlier, the strangely random variability of latency: see Sections 1.3 and 5.3), but a deliberate mechanism of procrastination. A possible early response is suppressed in order to decide more carefully on a later one. Because of this procrastination, latency is in effect telling us how long it takes the higher levels to decide what to look at. So what latency represents is the time needed to work out which of all the possible things we might do is best. *Reaction time is decision time.*

1.3 Analysing the Variability of Reaction Time

When you can measure what you are speaking about, and express it in numbers, you know something about it; but when you cannot measure it, when you cannot express it in numbers, your knowledge is of a meagre and unsatisfactory kind.
William Thomson, Lord Kelvin, "Electrical Units of Measurement" (1884)

When Nature does something odd, it is often a sign of a vulnerability asking to be scientifically exploited. With modern computer-based equipment, it is possible to obtain very large data sets of saccadic latency measurements and determine rather precisely the form of this random variability, as a first step to trying to understand why it happens.

It turns out that random reaction times obey a relatively simple law that applies not just to saccades to visual targets, but also to all kinds of responses, to a wide variety of stimuli, and in a remarkably similar way throughout the animal kingdom, from frogs to humans. A natural first step is to look at the distribution of variability across different trials in an experimental run, in the hope we can characterise the type of stochastic process that may be giving rise to it. Curiously enough, although some of the earliest experimenters were very well aware of the importance of doing this (Yerkes 1904), in general it has been rare for those who have measured reaction times to bother to publish more than means or medians of their data. Perhaps as a consequence, while many have developed more or less elaborate theories to relate *average* reaction times to stimulus or response parameters, rather few have been equally concerned with the *distribution* of the reaction times themselves (Noorani and Carpenter 2011, Antoniades and Carpenter 2012, Carpenter 2012). Of those who have, some have used them in half-hearted tests of models arrived at on theoretical grounds: some examples are presented in Appendix 1. Even Luce's masterly analysis (Luce 1986) of a wide range of models for reaction times devotes relatively little space to the critical evaluation of such models against existing distributional data. It almost begs belief that in so many experiments, particularly in the clinical arena, this information is simply thrown away (Antoniades and Carpenter 2012, Carpenter 2012).

The particular reaction time distribution that forms the focus of this book arose not theoretically but empirically, as the result of a search for some way of summarising large amounts of data from saccadic latencies. It was only subsequently that a very simple functional explanation for its existence was proposed (Carpenter 1981). The discovery that the same model seemed to underlie very many kinds of reaction time tasks, and provided a remarkably good fit to previously published distribution data from both early and recent sources, came relatively late. Thus, whereas the traditional approach has generally been to devise a good theory and only then (perhaps) see if it works, the novelty here was to start with an empirical description and find a theory for it later. Since the model has very few parameters and the theory is a simple one, the approach does not seem entirely unjustified. In the circumstances, it would be surprising if the nature of this distribution had never occurred to anyone before. Yet apart from a passing mention by Jenkins (1926) in a list of theoretical possibilities (if indeed that is what he meant by a 'harmonic' distribution), this appears to be the case.

1.3.1 Kinds of Histograms

The conventional way of presenting data about stochastic distributions is the frequency histogram. We start by dividing the range of possible data values into a series of 'bins' (or categories), usually of equal width. For reaction times, which usually range from a few tens to several hundred milliseconds, 10 ms is quite a convenient choice of bin-width. We then take each of our data values and assign it to a corresponding bin, keeping a tally of how many end up in each one. The result is then typically plotted as a bar chart (Figure 1.9).

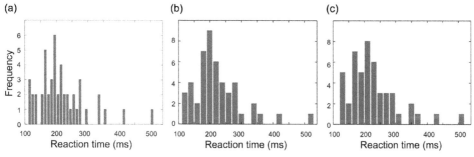

Figure 1.9 The arbitrariness of frequency histograms. The same data set (*N* = 50) is plotted first with 10 ms bins (a), then with 20 ms bins (b), and finally (c) with the 20 ms bins shifted by 10 ms.

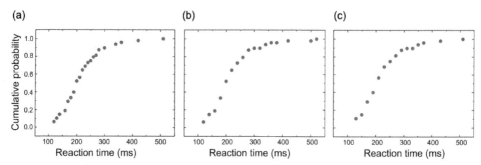

Figure 1.10 The same histograms as shown in Figure 1.9, but plotted cumulatively (a,b,c): their shapes are essentially unaffected by bin size or displacement.

Histograms of this kind are familiar and intuitive, but suffer from a number of grave defects: from a mathematical point of view, they are thoroughly unsatisfactory. Unless the data set is extremely large, they have randomly bumpy profiles that can give rise to spurious conclusions about the form of the data. Furthermore, the position and size of these bumps depend on what bin-width one happens to have chosen and where their boundaries are (Figure 1.9). In addition, the Y-axis of a frequency histogram is arbitrary: it too depends both on the width of the bins and on the total number of data points, making it difficult to make a visual comparison between one set of data and another. Finally, it is not easy to present several different frequency histograms in the same chart, so they are wasteful of space.

Fortunately, there is another way of plotting distributional data that solves all of these problems: the cumulative histogram. Here, instead of asking 'How many data points lie between 200 and 210 ms? How many between 210 and 220?' and so on, we ask a simpler question: 'How many are less than 210 ms? How many less than 220?' The result (Figure 1.10) is a curve that necessarily increases to the right, and is normalised in the sense that it must start at zero (there will always be *some* x value smaller than any of the data) and finish at 100% (since there must similarly be *an* x value that is bigger than all the data). If we choose to plot percentages rather than raw numbers, then this cumulative histogram is automatically normalised. Bin-width no longer has any effect on the overall shape; it simply alters the resolution, so that the arbitrariness of the appearance of the frequency histogram is avoided. Finally, we can have several cumulative histograms on one chart without confusion (Figure 1.11).

One kind of distribution that crops up again and again in scientific work is the Gaussian or Normal distribution (Gauss 1809) – popularly known as the 'bell curve'. It is the most fundamental of all random distributions, since mathematically it results from any situation in which a very large number of independent random events – which need not themselves be Gaussian – add together in a linear fashion. It is not surprising that much biological variation is Gaussian, since it results from the summation of a multiplicity of tiny genetic and environmental factors. Plotted as a conventional frequency distribution, it is indeed bell-shaped (Figure 1.12). To specify its shape, we need only two parameters: the mean (μ) and the standard deviation (σ). Often it is convenient to refer to the variance, σ^2.

If we are applying this to frequency distributions, it can also be referred to as the probability density function or PDF, $P(Z)$. The formula for P is given in Appendix 1,

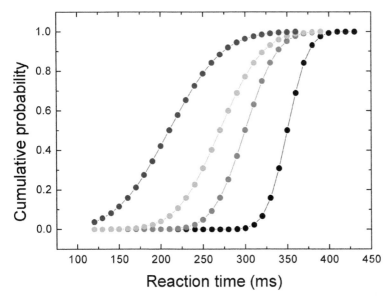

Figure 1.11 Several cumulative histograms can be shown in one graphic.

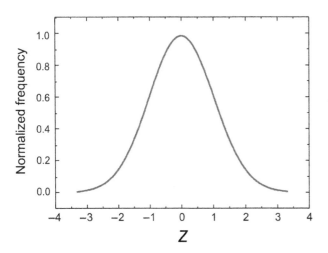

Figure 1.12 Gaussian frequency function, normalised to have a value of 1 at the mean, μ (in this case, zero). The horizontal Z scale (X-axis) shows deviations of x from the mean, in units of σ: so Z = 2 means that x is two standard deviations from the mean.

App 1.2. Corresponding to the PDF is its integral, the cumulative distribution function or CDF, $C(Z)$, whose formula is also given in Appendix 1, App 1.2. It is S-shaped (Figure 1.13) and is normalised in the sense that it ranges from 0 to 1.

Finally, there is a clever trick for seeing immediately whether a given distribution is or is not normal, which is not as well known generally as it ought to be. It is to plot a histogram using not a linear scale for the cumulative probability, but a distorted one (rather like log-paper) that is stretched out at both low and high probabilities in such a way as to turn the S-shaped distribution into a straight line. More specifically, this is a probit or 'probability' scale, that simply embodies the inverse of equation (2) above; distances Z along it can be thought of in units of one standard deviation, with zero in the

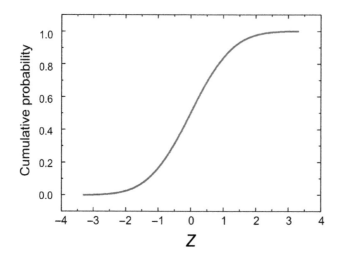

Figure 1.13 The same Gaussian function as in Figure 1.11, plotted cumulatively as the CDF, C(Z).

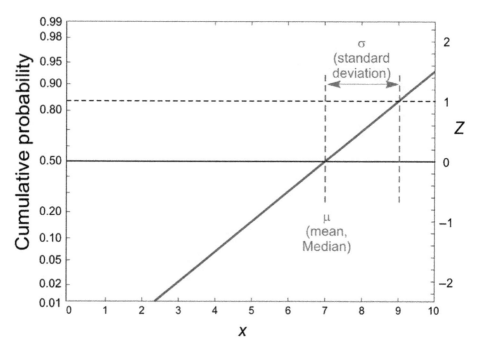

Figure 1.14 A normal distribution plotted cumulatively using a probit scale generates a straight line.

middle (corresponding to the mean or median, $C = 50\%$; thus, $Z = 1$ corresponds to 1 standard deviation (SD) from the mean, or $P = 84.1\%$; $Z = 2$ is the same as $P = 97.7\%$, and so on).

If the distribution in question is indeed Gaussian, its parameters can be derived directly from this straight line. The mean (and median) is the value of x where the line cuts the horizontal line at $C = 0.5$; the slope of the line is inversely related to σ (Figure 1.14). More exactly, σ is given by the horizontal distance between where the line intercepts $C = 0.5$ and where it intercepts $Z = 1$.

1.4 The Recinormal Distribution

Now conventional histograms of reaction times are not Gaussian, or even symmetrical. They have a long tail that extends further in the direction of long reaction times than short. This is a nuisance: the distribution does not fit any of the more standard mathematical distributions (Gaussian, Poisson, Gamma, etc.) particularly well. A lot of fruitless effort culminated finally in the realisation that the lack of success was simply an indication that one was thinking about the problem the wrong way.

Because we measure reaction times using clocks or their computer equivalents, which tick away in a linear fashion, it is natural to assume that the time taken to respond is a fundamental variable. But if we ask, instead, not about how the response is *measured* but how it is *generated*, we come to a completely different conclusion. Think, for instance, of a process initiated by the stimulus and proceeding at a certain rate until some criterion is reached that completes the decision and initiates a response. If there is variability in the time that is taken, isn't the simplest explanation that the rate at which the process occurs is varying? This is what we see in chemical reactions, for instance, if we vary the temperature. So instead of looking at reaction *times* (T), we should be looking at reaction *rates*: we should be analysing not T, but $1/T$, the reciprocal of the reaction time, or *promptness*.

Suppose, then, we create a conventional histogram not of reaction time but of promptness. We could do this with a computer, but in some ways it's more fun to use a graphical technique that lets us see what is going on more directly. The trick is to use a special scale – a reciprocal scale – that transforms distances into their reciprocals, just as the more familiar log scale does for logarithms. To aid interpretation, longer times are still to the right, and it's convenient to have our 'origin' (actually equivalent to infinity, since $1/T$ is then zero) to the right. Here's the result (Figure 1.15). Magically, we suddenly find that the asymmetry that is such an awkward feature of conventional plots has disappeared – indeed, the histogram looks Gaussian. This not only makes for easier mathematical analysis, but also suggests that we have reached a genuinely fundamental phenomenon.

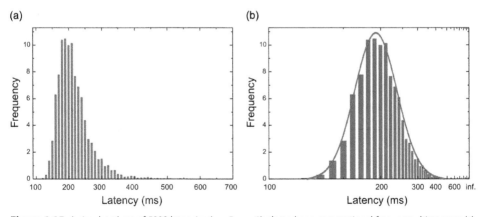

Figure 1.15 A simulated set of 5000 latencies ($\mu = 5$, $\sigma = 1$) plotted as a conventional frequency histogram (a), showing the obvious skewness of the distribution. (b) The same data plotted using a reciprocal sale for latency: note that for convenience the latencies still increase to the right. The distribution is now relatively symmetrical, and indeed very similar to a Gaussian (blue).

1.4.1 Reciprobit Plots

A convenient way to see at once whether reciprocal latency really is Gaussian is to use the trick described earlier (Section 1.3.1), of plotting latency as a cumulative histogram on a reciprocal scale. Then we repeat our trick of using a specially distorted scale, but this time on the vertical probability axis. This is a probit scale, specifically designed to stretch out the tails of the distribution in such a way that if the distribution is indeed Gaussian, we should get a straight line. Because it combines a reciprocal and a probit scale, we can call it a *reciprobit plot*. A Gaussian distribution of promptness should then give a straight line (Figure 1.16). The line intercepts the right-hand axis (t = infinity) at $Z = k$, given by μ/σ. It is also convenient to call the associated distribution a *recinormal distribution*. With certain reservations (Section 2.2), distributions of reaction times – not just for saccades but for other kinds of response as well – do indeed turn out to be recinormal.

On a reciprobit plot, the distribution cuts the horizontal 50% axis at the median: this is also the mean, since the distribution is Gaussian. Note that the intercept k represents a probability: that the linear approach to threshold ergodic rate (LATER) signal will never reach its threshold at all, in other words, that $r < 0$. Under most conditions, this probability is vanishingly small, but if we reduce the amount of available information, for instance by making discrimination increasingly difficult, this probability can be measured (see Section 4.7.2).

In Chapter 3, we introduce a simple model of a decision process that would give rise to such a distribution. Meanwhile, we need to separate clearly the purely empirical question of whether in fact real reaction times do or do not conform to a recinormal distribution, and what we can deduce about the underlying mechanisms if it turns out that they do. But

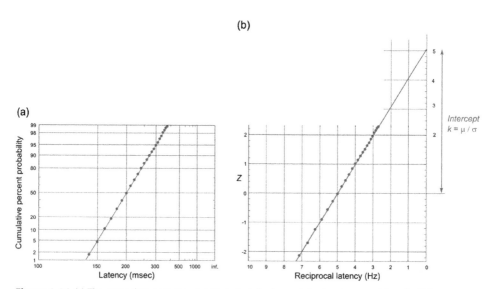

Figure 1.16 (a) The same data as in Figure 1.15, but plotted cumulatively using a probit scale. This systematically stretches the ends of the ordinate axis in such a way that if the data are indeed Gaussian, it generates a straight line. Since the latency uses a reciprocal scale, this is a reciprobit plot. (b) The same cumulative plot with the latency scale now explicitly of reciprocal latency (1/T), increasing leftwards to facilitate comparison; the probability scale uses units of Z. The data can be extrapolated to an intercept on the right-hand axis (T = infinity or 1/T = 0), whose value is μ/σ (in this case, 5) in Z units.

quite apart from the validity of any particular explanatory model, if it is true that sets of reaction times can be adequately described with only two parameters, this in itself has great practical importance, particularly in clinical studies (see Appendix 2).

1.4.2   A Gallery of Reciprobits

This observation on reaction times was originally discovered through analysis of saccadic data from our own laboratory. But to form some idea of its general applicability it seemed to us that a fairer and stricter test was to re-examine previously published data about latency distributions in as wide a range of situations as possible, and see whether they behaved the same way. What follows is a gallery of older data – published over the past hundred years or more – replotted as reciprobit plots. Kolmogorov–Smirnov (Kolmogorov 1941, Smirnov 1948) one-sample statistical tests are used to test conformity with a recinormal distribution, and none is significantly different ($p > 0.05$).

Figures 1.17–1.26 show reciprobit plots of 56 data sets taken from a wide cross section of the earlier published literature, covering a variety of types of response, of stimuli and of species. They are certainly not exhaustive; apart from omissions through ignorance, examples where the number of trials was too small (in general, fewer than 50) have been excluded, as have instances where the conditions of the experiment were insufficiently clearly described to be sure what it was that was being measured, or where data sets were needlessly repetitive. There is no wholly satisfactory way of arranging

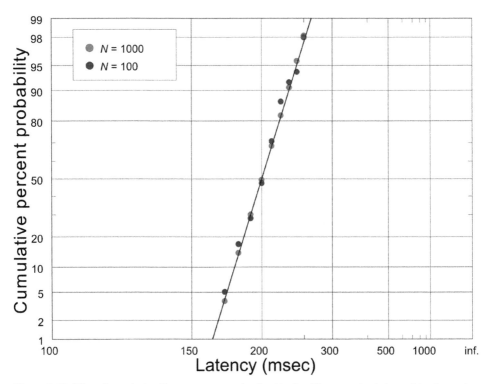

Figure 1.17 Effect of sample size, N, on appearance of reciprobit plots. These are simulations of simple reaction times with (left side of graph) N = 100, and (right side of graph) N = 1000.

them: we start with the relatively simple and finish with some more complex examples, and some that are frankly bizarre.

When comparing these plots, it is important to bear in mind two points.

The first is that because of the probit scale, in general these plots hugely exaggerate the extreme tails of the distribution. So the scatter which is the inevitable effect of random variation from trial to trial is very much more apparent at the two ends of the distribution than it is in the middle. In a large data set with a thousand measurements, the points in the region of 0.1% or 99.9% are derived from just one or two individual trials, and their exact position is consequently of little significance. As a result, we shall sometimes see that a distribution that fits a straight line very well in the centre may show quite substantial deviations at the ends despite being statistically perfectly acceptable. So distributions that are in fact absolutely compatible with a recinormal distribution may look poor to the unpractised eye because of a very small number of aberrant trials: the points at the extremes may only represent one or two individual trials: it is the points in the middle of the distribution that contribute most to goodness of fit.

Second, one must be aware of the overwhelming effect of the size N of a data set on the scatter of the points. With small data sets of a hundred or so, the apparent scatter will look much poorer than what is seen when N is a thousand or more (Figure 1.17), yet both may give equally good fits.

Finally, although most of the plots illustrate data sets for which essentially the entire population appears to conform to a recinormal distribution, in some there are examples of cases where there appears to be a small sub-population of unusually fast responses. In general, these early responses tend to lie along a different straight line that goes through what is in effect the origin of these reciprobit plots, namely, the intercept (t = infinity, C = 50%). They are considered in more detail in Section 2.2

We start with human saccadic responses to visual targets. Figure 1.18(a) gives an idea of how robust these distributions are over time. Though a little ragged because of the small N, the two runs happened to be made by the same subject with identical stimuli and conditions on two occasions separated by six years, and the two distributions are not statistically distinguishable (Kolmogorov–Smirnov (K-S) test (Kolmogorov 1941, Smirnov 1948)), giving some idea of the kind of stability that saccadic latencies can show under controlled conditions. Figure 18(b) and (c) show older data for saccades in a step task with variation of the eccentricity of the target (White, Eason et al. 1962), or its

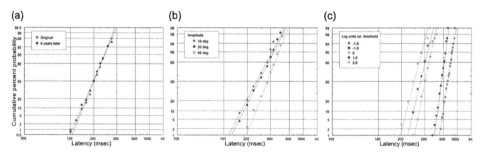

Figure 1.18 Reciprobit plots of human saccadic latencies to step targets. (a) Two different runs of around 100 trials at an interval of 6 years (R. H. S. Carpenter, unpublished data); (b) different amplitudes, 120 trials per data set (White, Eason et al. 1962); (c) different target luminances, expressed in log units relative to foveal threshold, 100 trials per data set (Wheeless, Cohen et al. 1967);

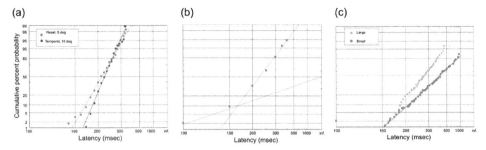

Figure 1.19 Other species. (a) Monkey, nasal saccades with an amplitude of 5 deg (123 trials) and temporal saccades of 10 deg (89 trials); a K-S test shows that the difference between the plots is not statistically significant (Fuchs 1967). (b) Cat saccades, 95 trials, showing an early component (Evinger and Fuchs 1978). (c) Cat nose-poke responses, for trials with large and small rewards (Avila and Lin 2014).

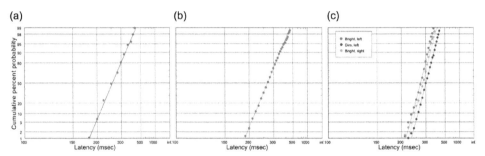

Figure 1.20 Manual human responses to visual stimuli. (a) From Walsh (1952); $N = 286$). (b) A large data set ($N = 825$) from a careful observer (Welford 1959). (c) From Johnson (1918), comparing left and right hands, and bright and dim stimuli; because of the large size of the data sets (ca. 900 trials each), the small difference between the left and right hands is in fact statistically significant (K-S test). Note that manual responses are in general slower than saccadic, and tend to lack early components.

luminance (Wheeless, Cohen et al. 1967). Despite the variation in the stimulus conditions (which in the latter case produce a variation in median latency by more than a factor of two), each data set conforms to the recinormal distribution. Changes in eccentricity appear to alter μ but leave k relatively unchanged, while target luminance seems to influence both.

Figure 1.19 shows responses in some other species: monkey, cat (with prominent early responses) together with nose-poke latencies in the rat.

Figures 1.20 and 1.21 show manual human responses mostly to visual stimuli, some with large data sets that demonstrate the extent to which in such cases the accuracy of the recinormality extends far into the tails of the distributions. They also include examples of experimental manipulation, for instance, by pharmacological substances.

Figure 1.22 shows manual responses to auditory stimuli. These data (McGill 1963, McGill and Gibbon 1965) have frequently been reproduced for the purpose of testing theories of reaction-time distribution, perhaps because they are both remarkably regular, considering their very small values of N. In both cases, the effect of reducing the stimulus intensity is to lengthen reaction times, the curves tending to swivel round a fixed value of k rather than simply being displaced to the right in a parallel fashion. One of the sets (40 decibels (dB)) is oddly bent, but otherwise the fits are very good.

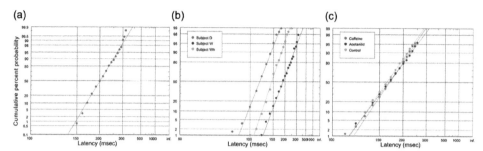

Figure 1.21 Manual human responses. (a) To visual stimuli (Schupp and Schlier 1972), instructive in that its statistical fit ($p = 0.91$, K-S test; $N = 546$) is much better than might be expected from its appearance, showing the importance of data points near the median as opposed to the tails. (b) Auditory, from three of Wells' subjects, D (194 trials), W (95) and Wh (196), two with a slight hint of an early component (Wells 1913). (c) Visual, from Schilling 1921, #3770, comparing the effects of two pharmacological substances, caffeine and acetanilide, with a control; in fact, the plots are not significantly different from one another (K-S test) despite the large data sets (800 trials each).

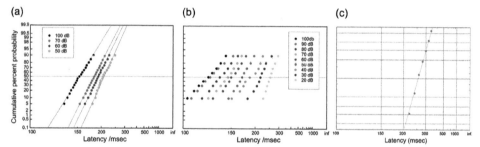

Figure 1.22 Manual reaction times to auditory stimuli of different intensities. (a) Human: 4 different intensities, 100 trials each (McGill and Gibbon 1965). (b) Human, 9 different intensities, 60 trials each (McGill 1963). (c) Cat manual responses (389 trials) to an auditory stimulus (Schmied, Benita et al. 1979).

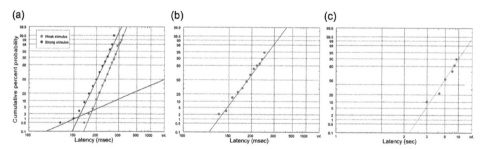

Figure 1.23 Some of the earliest distributions to be published. (a) Two of Kiesow's (Kiesow 1904) sets of reaction times to tactile stimuli of various strengths ($N = 200$), with a hint of an early component with the strong stimulus. (b) Frog reaction time to touch (Yerkes 1904). (c) The very long jellyfish reaction time to light, but a very small data set ($N = 10$): as a result, it is ragged, though not significantly different from recinormal (K-S test) (Yerkes 1903).

Finally, some extremely early data sets, dating from over a century ago (Figure 1.23). The Kiesow data are interesting (Figure 1.23(a)) in that they use a tactile stimulus, and also clearly demonstrate an effect of changing the strength of the stimulus. Figure 1.23(b) is also tactile, in a frog: it is ragged because of the small number of observations, but statistically

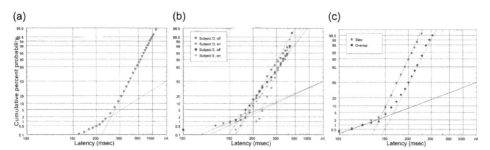

Figure 1.24 Human reaction times with prominent early components. (a) Manual auditory, 4436 trials (Green and Luce 1971). (b) Manual, two subjects, to illumination or extinction of visual target, 400 trials each (Jenkins 1926). (c) Saccadic, in step (red, 1875 trials) and overlap (blue, 998) tasks (Carpenter 1994).

compatible with a recinormal, as is the final even smaller data set (Figure 1.23(c)) showing the (very slow) responses of a jellyfish to light.

A graphical procedure like the reciprobit plot can often provide more insight than blind number-crunching. For instance, if you look critically at the Kiesow data, though the great majority of the blue data points lie satisfactorily on the expected straight line, the very earliest data point is much too high – there are more early responses than the law would predict. When we look at very large data sets (for example, Figure 1.23(a)), especially under conditions where the target is highly expected or the subject is trying as hard as possible to be fast, it is clear that there is indeed a separate sub-population of faster responses that lie on a different line, intersecting the main one but of shallower slope and extrapolating to the origin (the point corresponding to infinity and $p = 0.5$). Although these early responses look prominent on a reciprobit plot, they typically form only a small proportion of the population (some 2–5%) and therefore do not normally have a significant effect on the goodness of fit of the population as a whole (Section 2.2).

Figure 1.24 shows examples of distributions in which an early sub-population is more marked, though in no case do they form more than 2% of the total. Figure 1.24(a), of manual responses to an auditory stimulus (Green and Luce 1971), is a very large data set indeed ($N = 4436$); as a result, the shape of both the main population and the sub-population is particularly sharply defined. This is followed by plots of manual responses by two subjects to the illumination or extinction of a visual target (Figure 1.24(b)), with prominent early sub-populations, and finally human saccadic responses in a step and in an overlap task (Carpenter 1994) (Figure 1.24(c)), where the large value of n again results in a clear definition of the early sub-population. In each case, these early responses seem to lie on a straight line of much shallower slope than the main distribution that passes through $C = 50\%$ at $t = \infty$ (in other words, $\mu = 0$ and therefore $k = 0$). A model for these early responses is presented in Section 2.2.

1.4.3 But Are Saccades the Result of a Decision?

When we move our eyes to a suddenly presented target, is it reasonable to call it a decision? In ordinary parlance, we tend to use 'decision' to describe much more protracted processes: deciding to get out of bed, deciding what to have for breakfast, deciding where to go on holiday. Even pressing a button when a light comes on requires so little thought that it hardly seems appropriate to call it a decision at all, let alone the

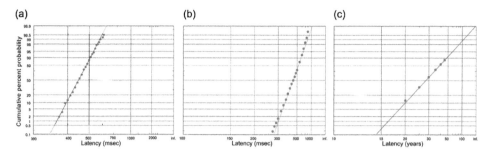

Figure 1.25 Some undeniable decisions. (a) In a task in which the subject had to decide whether the majority of a set of lines was inclined to the left or right (kind permission of Dr Ben Pearson). (b) Subjects decided whether a suddenly presented picture did or did not have an animal in it; note that this is combined data from 9 subjects (Thorpe, Fize et al. 1996). (c) A very long decision: age at first marriage for UK males in 2005 (web data, UK Home Office).

almost reflex response with which we flick our eyes on to a sudden visual target. But when we examine the form of the distributions of reaction times for different kinds of tasks – those that most people would consider reflexive, and those they would consider voluntary and therefore genuine 'decisions' – we find the identical, recinormal form for all of them. Figure 1.25 shows some examples. We see reciprobit plots for a difficult task in which the subject was presented with a set of lines of different orientations, and had to decide whether the majority were pointing in one direction rather than another (Figure 1.25(a)). The demanding nature of the task is reflected in the long mean reaction time (some 450 ms), but the form of the distribution is the same straight line that is seen in a saccadic step task. Figure 1.25(b) shows a large data set from (Thorpe, Fize et al. 1996) of the distribution of response times in a task that by any standards must be regarded as a 'decision': subjects had to respond to a picture of a complex scene by identifying whether or not it contained an animal. Because of the difficulty of the decision, the median reaction time is much longer; but – despite the degrading effect of combining data from several subjects – the recinormal law is still followed.

Finally, a very long decision indeed: Figure 1.25(c) shows the age at first marriage in the UK, and – very surprisingly – it follows the same recinormal distribution extremely well, despite the huge size ($N = 170,890!$) of the data set. Obviously, it is highly unlikely that this is due to the same neural mechanism giving rise to button-pushes and saccades, but the common principle is a process that reaches completion at a rate that is subject to Gaussian random variability which still applies.

1.4.4 Smooth Pursuit

We have seen that a visual target that suddenly appears, or jumps to a new position, typically evokes a saccade to fixate it. But when a target moves relatively smoothly and slowly, a completely different kind of eye movement is generated, called smooth pursuit (Rashbass 1961, Robinson, Gordon et al. 1986, Missal and Keller 2002, Thier and Ilg 2005). Whereas the function of the saccade is to capture a new target by moving it on to the fovea, smooth pursuit is intended to hold it there despite its movement. Like saccades, smooth pursuit is controlled by a sophisticated and intelligent system that does its best to anticipate how the target is going to move. As a result, the performance of a subject tracking a target that moves repetitively back and forth tends to get better and

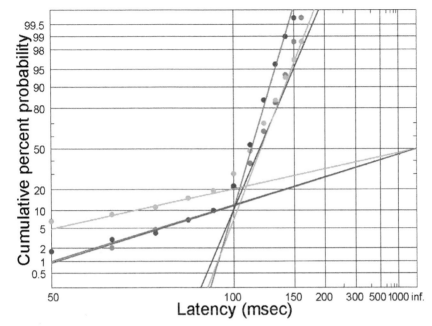

Figure 1.26 Initiation of smooth pursuit in response to a target moving off at constant velocity; 3 subjects, 300 trials each (Merrison and Carpenter 1995) showing prominent early responses.

better as time goes on and the brain is able to predict the motion. Figure 1.26 shows latencies of smooth pursuit by three subjects to a target suddenly moving off at constant velocity (Merrison and Carpenter 1995). Though these responses have a very short median latency, the general shape conforms very well to the pattern of the previous data sets, but with a much larger (10–20%) proportion of responses in the early sub-population. A saccade is usually made in each trial at about the same time as the smooth pursuit begins, intended to make up for the time lost during the latent period, during which the target has been moving (Rashbass 1961). It is quite interesting that the latencies of the smooth pursuit and saccadic responses in this situation are usually uncorrelated with each other, suggesting that there are separate units, acting independently, for saccades and smooth pursuit (Merrison and Carpenter 1994).

To summarise, reciprocals of reaction times are in general Gaussian. For data sets that are large enough to provide an adequate comparison, and if we ignore the existence of a small population of early responses, the recinormal distribution provides a better description than any other previously proposed, except in the case of distribution functions where the large number of parameters permits the function to be moulded, in effect, into the same shape as the recinormal (see Appendix 1, App 1.3–1.5). It is also clear that data sets of fewer than a hundred or so observations are of very little help in trying to validate theories of reaction time distributions. Unless a model is hopelessly inadequate, it will differ from other models only in the tails of the distribution: this is why we need large numbers of trials to evaluate one model decisively against another.

LATER as a Model of Latency

Nessuna certezza delle scientie è, dove no si può applicare una delle scientie matematiche e che non sono unite con esse matematiche.

No knowledge can be certain, if it is not capable of mathematical analysis, nor based on mathematics.
Leonardo da Vinci, Notebook *(1998)*

The fact that a large data set can be summarised with just two or three parameters is useful in itself – for instance, if we want to characterise clinical observations (examples of this are given in Appendix 2). But it is obviously not a factor that will drive evolutionary change. So why do reciprocals of reaction times have a normal distribution? What sort of mechanism could account for a recinormal distribution of latency? Does it make any functional sense? The model that is about to be presented was first conceived in relation to saccadic latencies (Carpenter 1981, 1988), but appears to have a much wider applicability. It will now be described briefly and then considered in more detail.

2.1 Linear Rise-to-Threshold

Earlier, we saw that the idea of analysing reciprocal latency follows from treating reaction time as the result of a process whose *rate* varies randomly from trial to trial.

Imagine a stimulus occurring at time zero. Let us suppose that its onset causes a decision signal S to rise linearly at a rate r from its initial value of S_0; and that when this signal reaches a predetermined threshold level S_T, a response is immediately initiated (Figure 2.1). The time elapsing between stimulus and response is the latency, T; it is convenient to designate the total rise of S, $(S_T - S_0)$, as θ, so it follows that $\theta = rT$. Though r is constant for any one trial, its value on different trials varies randomly with a Gaussian distribution having a mean μ_r and standard deviation σ_r. The reciprocal, s, of the latency will then be given by r/θ. Since r is distributed normally, so will s, with mean $\mu = \mu_r/\theta$ and standard deviation $\sigma = \sigma_r/\theta$. In other words, its distribution will be Gaussian, as in Figure 2.1, while the resultant distribution of the latencies themselves will show the skewness characteristic of reaction times. This is the LATER model (an acronym – Linear Approach to Threshold with Ergodic Rate – that also reminds one of the procrastination that it describes). Note that in LATER there is always a finite probability that $r < 0$, in which case the threshold is never reached.

The three parameters of the model (μ_r, σ_r, and θ) are intimately related to the three salient features of a reciprobit plot (slope, median, and intercept). Changes of the mean rate of rise, μ_r, move the reciprobit line horizontally parallel to itself, altering the

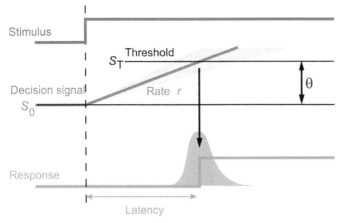

Figure 2.1 LATER model. A decision signal S whose initial value is S_0 begins to rise in response to the stimulus at a constant rate r until it reaches a threshold at $S_T = S_0 + \theta$, when it triggers the response. On different trials, r varies as a Gaussian with mean μ_r and variance σ_r^2; consequently, the latency distribution (green) is skewed.

intercept k but not the slope (Figure 2.2). On the other hand, changes in either S_0 or S_T, altering θ, will cause the line to swivel around the intercept k. The ratio of the mean and standard deviation of the population will remain constant, a feature noted by Chocholle (1940) as being common in reaction-time statistics under different experimental conditions. Finally, alterations in σ_r will cause the line to rotate about the median, which will remain fixed while the slope and intercept change. Evidently, LATER cannot as it stands be considered a very realistic representation of the actual mechanisms of latency in the body, for it takes no account of the physiological delays, mentioned earlier, that must intervene between the occurrence of the stimulus and the initiation of r, and between the arrival of S at S_T and the generation of the response. In fact, such delays are in practice small enough that their effects on the linearity of reciprobit plots of real data are negligible (Appendix 1, App 1.6.1) unless the data sets are extremely large, so for the moment they will be neglected.

Reciprobit plots obtained under different conditions can give one an immediate idea of how these conditions affect the model. However, some caution is needed, since of the three parameters (μ_r, σ_r, and θ) only two are independent. Although the obvious, and most economical, interpretation of a parallel shift of a reciprobit plot is a change in μ_r alone, strictly speaking, it could equally be explained by a simultaneous and equal proportional changes in both θ and σ_r, with μ remaining constant. As always, there is a degree of conflict between a model with many parameters, that must inevitably fit observed data better with one with fewer, and for this reason some authors (Nakahara, Nakamura et al. 2006, Brown and Heathcote 2008) have proposed adding a third independent parameter to LATER; but since two parameters already work well (Section 1.4.2) and provide a simple outcome for the purpose of clinical evaluation, there is little to be gained by adding another, in our opinion.

It is also true that in general there is often significant correlation between the latency for one trial and the next (Otto and Mamassian 2012), but it is not clear to what extent this is due to fluctuating prior probabilities, caused, for example, by the subject's expectation (Section 3.5) or by drowsiness or other global and slowly varying factors.

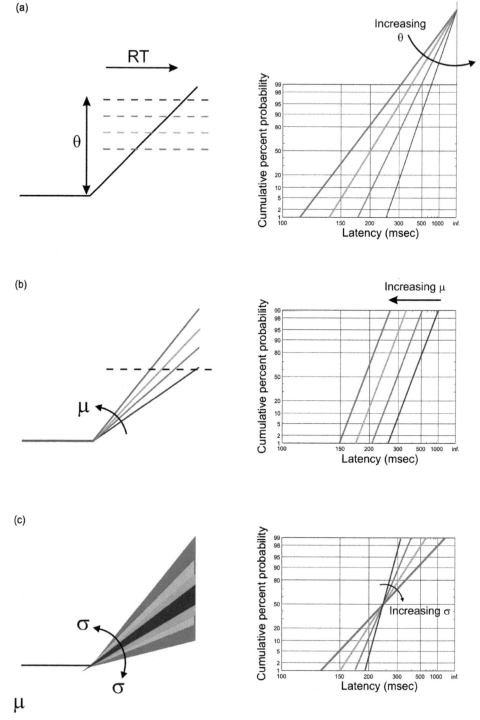

Figure 2.2 Relation between parameters of the model and of the reciprobit plot. (a) Variation in the threshold θ makes the plot swivel about the infinite intercept; (b) variation in the mean rate of rise μ leads to horizontal, self-parallel translation of the plot; (c) altering the variance σ_r^2 generates a change in the slope with no change in median latency. From Noorani and Carpenter (2016).

In addition, in more complex tasks there are likely to be shorter-term consequences of the immediately preceding trial that are also likely to generate correlations (Fecteau and Munoz 2003, Tatler and Hutton 2006).

In the real world, when there are many stimuli competing for our attention, we can envisage a number of LATER units operating in parallel and racing against one another, with the winner initiating its associated response. One can imagine that these multiple units also sharpen the competition through mechanisms of lateral inhibition of the kind that has been demonstrated between saccadic target-selecting units in frontal cortex (Schall and Hanes 1993); this is discussed further in Section 4.4.

2.2 Early Responses

In the early days of cerebral physiology when functions were first localised in 'centres' in the cortex of the brain it was assumed that the only duty of these 'centres' was to bring about various reactions of the body in response to its needs or to its environment when acting under the influence of consciousness, or 'will', whatever it may be; but modern work has emphasised that they are largely concerned in keeping subcortical activities under proper control. The higher centres can be, in fact, compared to the second chamber of a legislature which is capable of action on its own, but its chief function is to prevent an assembly representative of many and diverse interests, but less well informed of all the bearings and facts of the situation and, therefore, less discriminative, from reacting to every impulse of the moment.
Gordon Holmes, 'Looking and Seeing' (1936)

Some of the distributions of Figures 1.17–1.26 in Chapter 1 show a feature that cannot be explained in terms of a single LATER unit: an additional small population of short-latency responses that produces a deviation from the expected straight line. These *early responses* may include, but are not synonymous with, what are commonly called 'express saccades' (Section 2.2.2). The difference is that true express saccades form a genuinely bimodal population, whereas the population of early saccades typically overlaps the main distribution with no distinct mode of its own, and is only easily perceived when a reciprobit plot is used. This second population of early responses usually lies along a second straight line, representing a recinormal distribution with $k = 0$ and a shallower slope that corresponds to a σ three or four times the typical values seen in the main part of the distribution (Figure 2.3). It is convenient to call this standard deviation σ_E.

Though easily visible in a reciprobit plot, such responses typically only represent some 3% of the total. As result, their distribution is not easily characterised unless we have something like the huge data set shown in Figure 1.24(a). In addition, the two mechanisms seem to show a degree of independence: in Figure 1.24(c), the early line remains fixed despite a shift of some 30 ms in the main response line under the two conditions. But this is not always the case: sometimes the early response line is flatter and sometimes steeper, altering the proportion of early responses to the whole in different circumstances, and its slope may be correlated with that of the main distribution (see Chapter 3, Figure 3.7). With targets that are unexpected, the proportion decreases; when the target is anticipated by the subject, either because of a prior cue, such as extinction of a fixation spot before the target appears, or by increasing the proportion of trials on which a particular target occurs, the proportion increases substantially and may reach as much as 10% (Carpenter and Williams 1995). 'Cognitive' distraction (Halliday and

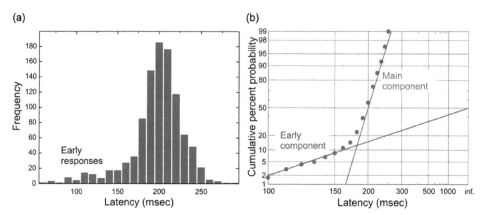

Figure 2.3 A distribution with a prominent early component. (a) Its frequency histogram. (b) Reciprobit plot: the lines correspond to the best-fit main (blue) and early (red) recinormal components. From Noorani and Carpenter (2016).

Carpenter 2010) can also greatly increase the number of early responses, as does instructions to the subject to be as fast as possible and not worry about mistakes: possible mechanisms of these effects are discussed in Section 3.6.

This suggests that what we need is two LATER units in parallel, one having a relatively large μ and small σ, and generating the main part of the distribution, and the other having a much larger value of σ but with μ equal to zero. Usually this second 'maverick' unit is overtaken by the main unit, so that most responses lie on the main part of the distribution. But just occasionally the large σ of the maverick unit causes it to overtake the main one, generating an aberrantly early response. It is tempting to identify the main unit with higher, cortical levels of the system and the maverick unit with the superior collicular level, normally suppressed by the descending tonic inhibition described earlier. We shall see later that both urgency and increased expectation tend to increase the number of early responses. Monte-Carlo simulations – using randomly chosen parameters on each trial – generate distributions that are very similar to what is observed in practice. Once a model has more than one LATER unit, analytical solutions may be difficult or impossible to discover. One example of an analytical solution for a combination of two competing units can be found in Appendix 1, App 1.8.2 and Noorani and Carpenter (2016) – but, in general, analytical models are difficult to generate, whereas stochastic simulations are perfectly adequate, and we can have as many iterations as we need to achieve any desired accuracy. By seeing them actually running, one may gain greater insight into their function (Figure 2.4).

Another possibility for modelling the maverick unit would be to use a Poisson process (see Appendix 1, App 1.5.1) with a constant probability per unit time of making an early response; this might seem plausible, but it produces plots that do not extrapolate back to $C = 50\%$ at infinite time. Finally, it is important to point out that although for clarity it can often be helpful to plot the asymptotes – in effect, the two separate components corresponding to the main and maverick components – the data points will not be expected to go through them: an alternative is to plot the combined theoretical distribution resulting from both components together (Figure 2.5)

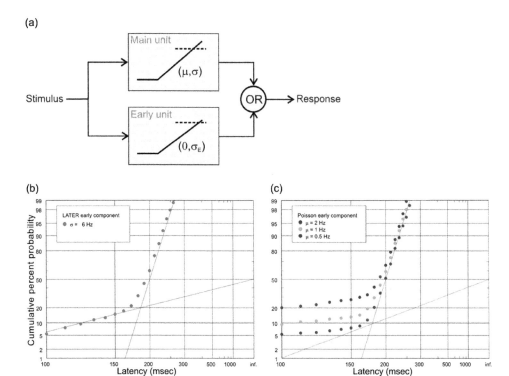

Figure 2.4 Modelling the early component, (a) A main unit with parameters μ and σ operates in parallel with a 'maverick' early unit (parameters $\mu = 0$ and σ_E.) The response is triggered by whichever unit reaches threshold first. Recinormal and Poisson early components: simulations with 1000 trials each. A recinormal distribution in parallel with (b) another recinormal having $\mu = 0$ and $\sigma_E = 6$; (c) three Poisson distributions with the rate parameters shown. The lines are separate main and early components (best-fit in (b)): in (c), it can be seen that the Poisson early components do not in general have the property of extrapolating back to the origin, characteristic of actual data.

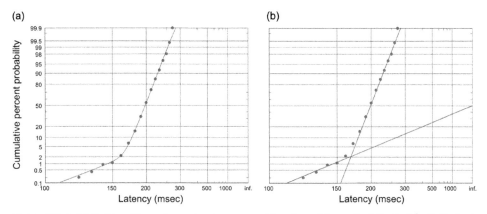

Figure 2.5 A distribution with a recinormal early component ($\mu = 5$, $\sigma = 0.5$, $\sigma_E = 3$) plotted in (a) with the best-fit theoretical line, and in (b) with just the asymptotes of the two theoretical components: note that in general the latter will not actually go through all the data points.

2.2.1 Multiple Early Units

We shall see in Section 4.8 that the intervals between saccades during spontaneous scanning share many of the stochastic properties of evoked latencies and are almost certainly due to the same underlying LATER mechanism. They tend to have particularly large early components, which may sometimes not extrapolate to $k = 0$ but to a higher value. They can often be modelled by having multiple early units in parallel, as shown in Figure 2.6(a), perhaps corresponding to an increased number of potential targets that could attract early responses. The resulting distributions have increasing k-values with increasing numbers of units (Figure 2.6(b)): more exactly, the equivalent cumulative intercept probabilities are given by $(1 - 0.5^n)$, where n is the number of early units. Some examples relating to reading are shown in Figure 4.22 in Chapter 4, where the number of early units seems to be in the range 3–5.

2.2.2 Express Responses

In the case of saccades, the identification of these early responses is complicated by the existence of a different sub-population of faster responses, the *express* saccades first described by Fischer and Boch (1983) and Fischer and Ramsperger (1984), with which the early responses are often confused in the literature. These too form a population that is distinct from the main group, but with an important difference. Rather than lying on a separate straight line through the origin, they typically form a separate peak in the raw histogram, usually resulting in a bimodal distribution that can be recognised at once in reciprobit plots; that they are distinct from the early responses is clear from cases in which both components can be seen at once. The whole area of express responses has been thoroughly reviewed by Fischer and Weber, who propose a model in which a pre-emptive random choice is made on each trial, between pathways embodying different delays (Fischer and Boch 1983, 1984, Fischer and Ramsperger 1984, Fischer and Weber 1993, Fischer, Weber et al. 1993, Fischer, Geleck et al. 1995), the shorter being perhaps collicular and the longer cortical delay (Beck, Ma et al. 2008) (Figure 2.7). The mechanism of express saccades is further discussed in Appendix 1, App 1.8.1.

Finally, another subset of *late* responses can sometimes be seen, which lengthens the distribution to the right. Like express saccades, late saccades may also produce a bimodal distribution. Almost always, they are caused by inattention or drowsiness.

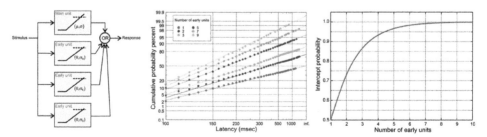

Figure 2.6 (a) Multiple early units in parallel with a main LATER unit. (b) Simulations of distributions for different numbers of early units, each with $\sigma_E = 5$, as shown: for clarity, the early components are shown on their own with no main unit, and each distribution represents 2000 trials. (c) The relationship between the number of early units and the probability corresponding to the intercept.

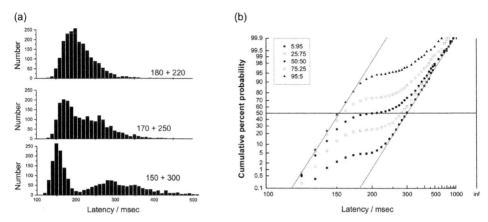

Figure 2.7 Express responses. Results of simulations ($N = 2047$) of a model in which one of a pair of recinormal processes is chosen at random on each trial. (a) Raw histograms for the case when the recinormals are chosen with equal frequency and have identical values of $k = 7$, but different pairs of values of median latency: 180 and 220 ms, 170 and 250, or 150 and 300. (b) Reciprobit plots of the distributions shown on the left. The red lines show the expected distributions for the individual components on their own.

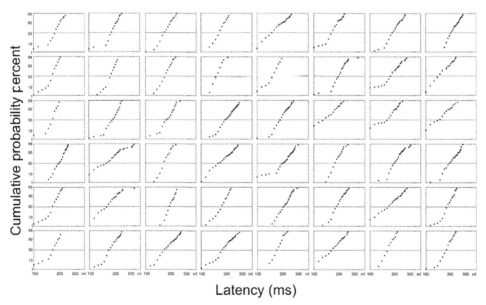

Figure 2.8 Reciprobits plots for a simple step task (200 trials) in 48 students of similar age and academic attainment, showing the considerable degree of variation between subjects in the main distribution and also in the incidence of early, express and late responses (Carpenter 2012).

Figure 2.8 shows a representative set of saccadic reciprobit plots over a population of students roughly matched for age and academic attainment, to give some idea of the variation typically seen both in the parameters of the main part of the distribution and in the incidence of early, express and late components.

(a) (b)

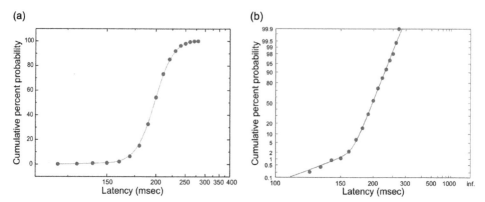

Figure 2.9 A distribution with an early component that can barely be discerned using a linear cumulative scale (a). But on a reciprobit plot (b) its characteristics are obvious). From Noorani and Carpenter (2016).

Finally, another powerful reason for using reciprobits is that early responses are often virtually invisible on cumulative plots using a linear probability scale, even with a reciprocal time axis (Figure 2.9); worse still is the pernicious technique of quintiling (Noorani and Carpenter 2011), in which only the middle of the distribution is presented.

At present, much information is often thrown away by publishing only mean latencies and ignoring distributions (Noorani and Carpenter 2011, Antoniades and Carpenter 2012, Carpenter 2012). Since LATER is entirely described by just two parameters, from a purely pragmatic point of view, it provides an economical way of providing a complete description of reaction-time distribution data. This is particularly useful in clinical situations, where differences in saccadic latencies in particular are increasingly being used for the differential diagnosis of neurological conditions (Nettelbeck 1980, Pirozzolo and Hansch 1981, Hershey, Whicker et al. 1983, Makert and Flechtner 1989). Appendix 2 provides a summary of studies of this type. However, the huge variation over the population that is evident in Figure 2.8 also means that a single analysis of distribution in a patient can seldom provide reliable diagnostic evidence. Ideally, we want longitudinal data, comparing the parameters under different conditions in the same patient before and after trauma, for instance, or in evaluating the effectiveness of therapeutic procedures. This important point is discussed further in Appendix 2.

2.3 Manual Responses

In a typical simple manual reaction-time task, a subject presses a button in response to a visual or auditory stimulus. There is a fundamental difference here from a visual saccadic task: the relation between the stimulus and response is essentially *arbitrary*. A visually directed saccade is in a sense hard-wired, and we saw in Section 1.2 that in the superior colliculus in particular there are relatively primitive neural circuits that automatically map visual space on to saccadic space. But in the case of manual responses, there is no intrinsic logic in, say, pressing a button with the right hand when a light appears on the right, or the left hand when it is on the left. The subject must be instructed what to do, and could equally easily perform the opposite task, generating a left-hand response to a right-hand stimulus. This process of translation must take time, which no doubt contributes to the fact that manual reaction times are about 80 ms longer in young adults than

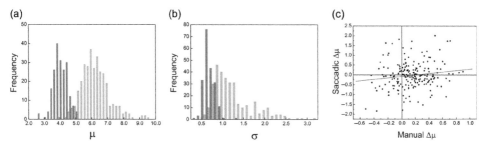

Figure 2.10 A comparison of manual (red) and saccadic (green) reaction times in a population of students. (a) Values of μ and (b) of σ. It is clear that manual reaction times are longer, but saccadic reaction time is more variable ($N = 321$ for the saccades, 200 for the manual data). (c) Manual and saccadic latencies are not significantly correlated across the population: the red regression line has $p = 0.88$. (Carpenter, unpublished data.)

saccades to the same stimulus (Figure 2.10). In addition, on the whole manual responses do not generate early responses: again, this may be due to the lack of a relatively automatic mechanism linking the stimulus and response. In this study, whereas 47% of the subjects showed an early component in their saccadic responses, only 23% did so in the manual task.

In other words, the mapping in this case is not intrinsic but must be programmed, which may be why little correlation is found between prowess at fast games, such as table tennis, and saccadic latency in the step task. With more complex situations (batting in cricket, for instance), it seems the oculomotor system can use quite subtle cues to improve its internal models (Land 1995, Land, Mennie et al. 1999, Land and McLeod 2000, Lenoir, Crevits et al. 2000a, 2000b, Land and Tatler 2009).

LATER as a Model of Decision

3

It is remarkable that a science which began with the consideration of games of chance should have become the most important object of human knowledge. . . . The most important questions of life are, for the most part, really only problems of probability.
Pierre Simon Laplace, Théorie analytique des probabilités *(1812)*

There are fashions in science just as in everything else, and the popularity of measuring the time required to make a response to a stimulus has waxed and waned over the years. The earliest investigators were motivated in part by a practical problem in astronomy, the difficulty of estimating the exact moment at which a star or planet reached the cross-hairs of a transit telescope (Wolf 1865, Mollon and Perkins 1996). This work revealed two striking kinds of variability. On average, different observers had very different reaction times (Henmon and Wells 1914) (the 'personal equation'); in addition, reaction times varied greatly from one occasion to another. Later, with the rise of quantitative psychophysics in the nineteenth century, reaction time came to be seen as an objective parameter of psychological perform-ance that could be obtained without very advanced recording technology (Boring 1929). But these data proved easier to obtain than to explain, and reaction times fell out of favour.

In the 1960s, interest revived once more as a consequence of the development of information theory, which amongst other things provided a theoretical framework into which such observations might be fitted (Luce 1959, Laming 1968, Welford 1980). But once the limits to the applicability of information theory in general became apparent, interest in reaction times similarly declined once again. What has led to a revival of interest in the past decade or two has been the realisation that reaction time provides a highly quantitative means of studying the neural mechanisms of *decision* (Schall 2000, Schall 2003, Shadlen and Gold 2004, Schall 2005, Gold and Shadlen 2007), itself an increasingly popular area of study, thanks in part to the rise of the remunerative but not notably successful field of neuroeconomics (Smith, Dickhaut et al. 2002, Glimcher and Rusticini 2004, Glimcher 2008, Platt and Huettel 2008).

Most experimenters, whether in the recent or more distant past, have been most interested in trying to relate the time taken to respond to a stimulus to aspects of the stimulus itself, or of the response. Difficult discriminations or complex actions lengthen reaction times, and responses to expected stimuli occur sooner than responses to unexpected ones. But an intrinsic feature of reaction times that also merits attention is their extraordinary *randomness*. With responses to target steps, remarkably stereotyped in every other respect, typically we find that with a mean of 200 ms, in 10% of trials the latency exceeds the range 160–260 ms.

In physiological terms, it is strange that there should be any variability at all. If reaction times were simply due to the time it takes for information to travel from receptors to muscles through the intervening nerves and synapses, its variability ought to be, if anything, rather less than the variability in conduction velocity or synaptic delay that is actually found in the laboratory. It is difficult to explain why, when all such factors are held strictly constant, the reaction time should be just as variable as ever. Has randomness evolved because it is actually beneficial in some way? Can one imagine decision mechanisms in which unpredictability is not an embarrassment, but inherent in the way the decision process operates? These important questions are discussed in Section 6.3.1.

For an experimenter who wishes to establish a causal relation between some external factor and reaction time, this variability is merely tiresome, since we have to average over large numbers of observations. But it must be telling us something important about the neural processes underlying the decision, and so is worth investigating in its own right.

3.1 An Ideal Decision-Maker

So far, LATER has been presented purely as a way of describing the distribution of reaction times. To be able to summarise data succinctly is something, but not much. A model that has no functional meaning is scarcely worthy of the name. Does LATER make any functional sense? It has already been argued that reaction time (mostly) represents decision time, so it is not unnatural to wonder whether the function of LATER is to make decisions. We might try turning the question round, asking instead what an ideal decision-making device ought to be like.

What exactly is a decision? In one sense, it is a commitment to a certain course of action, chosen from different alternative hypotheses – internal models of the real world – after consideration of relevant evidence. But this is a description of the final outcome, whereas – perhaps unfortunately – in common parlance we also use 'decision' to mean the entire process that leads up the final result. This is quite an important distinction, because although the final outcome is immutable, the process leading up to it is dominated by uncertainty. We may be uncertain about the evidence coming from our senses – was that really a tiger we just witnessed? More often, we are uncertain about the consequences of the different possible actions we might select – were those oysters really fresh? Biologically, everything we do costs energy that must be replaced; so, making a decision amounts to a gamble on whether the expenditure involved in the action will be more than repaid by the return we hope to get – like a company deciding whether the expected increase in profits justifies a new investment. In deciding whether to attack or not, the brain needs to form the best possible estimate of whether the energy expended is likely to be smaller or greater than the energy gained from eating the prey.

Decision-making therefore implies the calculation of *probabilities*.

3.2 What Is Probability?

The actual science of logic is conversant at present only with things certain, impossible or entirely doubtful, none of which (fortunately) we have to reason on. Therefore the true logic for this world is the calculus of probabilities, which takes account of the magnitude of the probability which is, or ought to be, in a reasonable man's mind.
James Clerk Maxwell, The Scientific Papers of James Clerk Maxwell
(Maxwell and Nivin 1890)

The simplest and most clear-cut problems in probability and decision arise in games of chance, and became a hugely popular area of study in early nineteenth-century Paris (Laplace 1812, Poisson 1837, Cournot 1843). Formally, the study of probability begins with what is called a *chance setup* – tossing a coin, throwing dice, drawing a lottery ball, spinning a roulette wheel – or any other situation in which we are uncertain about the outcome on any particular occasion or trial. In principle, we ought to be able to express this uncertainty numerically, and this is what we mean by the probability p: it is a measure of what we expect to happen. The equation $p = 1$ corresponds to absolute certainty that the event will happen, $p = 0$ to absolute certainty that it will not. What about in between? This has long been a contentious area, with different views often vehemently expressed (Venn 1876, Keynes 1921, Jeffreys 1939, Good 1959, Hacking 1965, Jeffrey 1965, Dempster 1968, Lucas 1970, Hacking 1975, Weatherford 1982, Shafer 1991, Lindley 2000, Howie 2002). Here we examine just five of them.

3.2.1 Frequency

Imagine a very long series of individual trials, for example of tossing a coin. Although we cannot say much about any particular trial, in the long run we can be increasingly confident about what will happen. If the coin is a fair one, then it should come down heads roughly half the time; the more trials we perform, the more we expect this ratio to converge to exactly 50%. This gives rise, naturally enough, to the *frequency* theory of probability (Venn 1876): we take p simply to be the proportion of trials which – in the very long term – the specified outcome is observed to occur. So we can say that the probability of getting heads is 0.5, of throwing a 6 with a die is 1/6, and so on. Building on this, we can derive rules for how probabilities combine. For instance, the probability of two independent events whose individual probabilities are p and q both occurring is given by ($p.q$).

This may all seem very reasonable: it is the version of probability usually taught in schools and generally adopted by physical scientists. But a little thought begins to make one uneasy about it. Do we really base our estimates of probability on observing very large numbers of trials? If someone tells us that a particular pack of cards has equal numbers of each suit, do we really have no idea what the probability is of drawing a diamond until we have tried a large number of times? When the UK National Lottery first began, were the designers completely in the dark about the probability of a given number being drawn?

3.2.2 Equipossibility

Imagine the first day of the brand-new UK National Lottery. There are 100 balls, identical apart from being numbered 1 to 100, and a blindfolded celebrity is to select 10 of them at random. Clearly, the cost of lottery tickets, and the value of the prizes, must be advertised in advance, so we need to know what the probability is of drawing any given set of 10 numbers. We consult an expert on probability, who happens to be a frequentist. '*But how can we possibly know what the probability is? Come back in a year's time when we have had a bit of experience of the thing and I can give you an answer.*' If we were to ask a physicist, however, we might get a more confident reply. Having satisfied himself that the balls really do lack any physical characteristic that would cause a blindfolded celebrity to choose one rather than another, he would argue that while we may not know from experience what is the probability of picking a particular ball, we do know (a) that this probability is the same for all of them, and (b) that the probability of picking some ball is 1. Therefore, we can deduce that the probability of picking any particular ball is 1/100. One solution is to use the principle of equipossibility: if there are, say, N outcomes, and there is no reason to expect one rather than another, then the probability of any particular outcome is $1/N$.

Equipossibility was used long before Venn's development of strict frequency theory as a way of estimating probabilities (Laplace 1812). If there are N possibilities, all equally likely, and the number of 'favourable' outcomes is M, then p is simply equal to M/N: 1/6 for throwing a 6 with a die, 1/2 for heads in a coin toss, 1/36 for a specified number on a roulette wheel with 36 holes, about 1 in 30 million for winning the top prize in the UK National Lottery. But we have now diverged completely from the idea of a series.

3.2.3 Propensity

We could also think of the lottery as a chance setup, a machine with an inbuilt propensity to generate random numbers with certain probabilities, so we do not need to observe a series of them to calculate what those probabilities must be. Nor do they have to be equal – the machine may be constructed (as fruit machines are) to generate some outcomes more often than others.

However, a moment's reflection shows that the realm of situations where the idea of propensity can be applied is very small, limited essentially entirely to human-made randomisers – roulette wheels and the like – specifically designed to generate random events with designated probabilities. It is also an appropriate way to think about the physics of systems with a large number of allegedly identical entities, such as electrons or the molecules in a gas. But real life is messy and complex: it is rare to have good grounds for asserting propensity, yet people have passionately held beliefs about the associated probabilities. Think of horse races, where each horse has can be regarded as having a certain propensity to win, but it is essentially impossible to calculate.

3.2.4 Logical Probability

A wholly different approach that avoids the difficulties inherent in trying to apply probability to the real world, either through frequency or propensity, is to treat probability as an essentially mathematical abstraction, a kind of generalisation and expansion of the established laws of logic. Conventional logic allows propositions only to be true or to be false, 1 or 0. But we can quite easily construct a formal logical system in which the truth of a proposition is allowed to be somewhere in between. Maynard Keynes (1921) created a mathematical framework that tells us how to manipulate such probabilities. Any conceptual scheme for probability must conform to such a structure if it is to behave rationally. Unfortunately, as with other beautiful self-contained mathematical constructs, what it does *not* do is show us how to discover what the probabilities of real events or hypotheses in the outside world actually are. Nor does it reflect the fact that different people typically have different ideas of the probability of any given event – were this not so, we would have no betting or bookmakers. But logical probability does at least ensure that statements about probabilities are self-consistent.

3.2.5 Subjective

Practical questions of the kind faced by insurance companies are even more problematic. Consider this question: What is the probability that I will die tomorrow? It is true that we could look at the frequency of dying for the entire world population. But of course the probability depends on one's age, on where one lives, on one's sex. As the series becomes more specific, it also becomes smaller: the probability must also depend on my lifestyle, on the fact that I don't drive and don't smoke, on my genetic inheritance, on my own medical history ... and in the end we have no series at all, just a single, unique individual!

Such considerations lead to a radically different view of probability: not as a frequency but as a measure (Good 1959) of subjective belief. This can include questions like *What is the probability of life on Mars?* – where people clearly have beliefs, despite there being no series of the kind required by the frequency theory, nor any possibility of estimating propensity. Or *What is the probability that the 100th decimal digit of π is 9?* Clearly the answer is completely determined; some people may happen to know the answer (it is in fact 9), and for them the probability is 1, but most will not, and for them (if they use equipossibility) it is likely to be 0.1. Variation in p from one person to another upsets many mathematicians, who are inclined to take the view that these erroneous subjective probabilities are just plain wrong. But a way of getting round this is to state that the value of p for a particular person must be correctly calculated from all the evidence that they have ever received. John Venn, not an advocate of subjective probability, wrote in 1876 (Venn 1876): ' ... *logic (and therefore probability as a branch of logic) is not concerned with what men do believe, but what they ought to believe, if they are to believe correctly'.*

Subjective probability tends to arouse particular hostility from the proponents of frequentism, to which it is perhaps least akin. As de Finetti observes (1937):

> *Two completely opposed points of view are possible: The first, the most commonly accepted, considers the subjective element of the naive notion of probability which is found in our everyday life as a dangerous element which ought to be eliminated in order that the notion of probability be able to attain a truly scientific status; the opposite point of view considers, on the contrary, that the subjective elements are essential, and cannot be eliminated without depriving the notion and theory of probability of all reason for existing. The difference between the two points of view is also very sharp from the philosophical point of view: according to the one, probability is an element which partakes of the physical world and exists outside of us; according to the other, it only expresses the opinion of an individual and cannot have meaning except in relation to him.*

Part of the problem is, I believe, a degree of misunderstanding about the implications of 'subjective'. For many scientists, this is a 'boo-word': it signifies unreliability, arbitrariness, and association with mystical stuff like 'consciousness'. But 'subjective' becomes 'objective' when instantiated in the neurons of the brain. These neurons are, after all, only machines; and it is in their interest to do a good job of computing probabilities: if they don't, we (and they) die. The same applies to robots driving cars. They too need to be able to compute probabilities, but these probabilities will also be subjective, since each car will have had different experiences. As Good has put it (1975): '*Even an intelligent robot would be advised to adopt a subjectivistic theory of probability and rationality, in the interest of self-preservation. More precisely, the robot, like a man, should behave as if he adopted these theories as an approximation.*'

3.2.6 Terminology

One thing that is apparent from all this is that the word 'probability' is over-worked and made to stand for many different things (see Appendix 1, App 1.1.2). This tends to generate ambiguity as well as animosity, which might be avoided if we were willing to be more specific in our terminology. Many others have felt the same, but unfortunately here too there has been a lack of unanimity. Peirce (1923) suggested using 'chance' and 'probability' to designate different things: *'Probability is the ratio of the favourable cases to all the cases. Instead of expressing our result in terms of this ratio, we may make use of another – the ratio of favourable to unfavourable cases. This last ratio may be called the chance of an event . . . (feeling of belief) should be as the logarithm of the chance'* (see Dale (1991). Peirce is advocating using 'probability' to include frequency, equipossibility, and propensity, with a more complex definition of chance. Nevertheless, it is clearer, I think, to use 'chance' solely to describe the probability of an *event*, and to reserve 'probability' for hypotheses and other propositions. But we have seen that probability can be regarded in at least three different ways. Perhaps one might reserve 'truth' for the most abstract and general formulation, of the Keynesian kind, and use 'credibility' to designate subjective belief; 'propensity' will probably do for propensity. 'Likelihood' is then a measure proportional to the probability of an event, contingent on some hypothesis, and like 'odds' it need not assume any particular interpretation of probability.

But we do of course need to agree that any interpretation of 'probability' yields values that range only from 0 to 1 – not true of odds, for instance, which can take any value from zero to infinity (Appendix 1, App 1.7.3). A further point, insisted on in particular by both Keynes (1921) and Nagel (1936), is that probability is a property of *relations* between propositions, not of the propositions themselves: we shall see later that this is precisely how the brain must encode probabilities. In fact, if the subjective (or neural) interpretation is admitted to hinge upon observed frequency to date, then some rapprochement between the different formulations is possible: Keynes (1921) remarked that chance is really a special case of subjective chance. Induction means calculating probabilities from events; deduction means calculating chances from hypotheses (limited, in logical deduction, to propositions for which $p = 0$ or 1).

3.2.7 Probability and Information

But different people have different experiences; so even if they all 'believe correctly', they will have different personal estimates of p. An important consequence of this subjective view of probability is the need to consider how in fact subject probabilities do – or should – change in the light of new evidence. If a friend throws a die on to a table, and it shows a 6 – but I don't look at it – for me the probability of it being a 6 is still 1/6. But when I turn round and see the actual result, the probability suddenly jumps to $p = 1$ (Figure 3.1). Why? Because I have received *information*. In fact, probability and information have a reciprocal relationship to each other: probability is a measure of uncertainty, or lack of information; conversely, we measure the amount of information we have received by the degree to which it changes our subjective probabilities. So, to understand decision-making we need to understand the relationship between probability and quantity of evidence. Like probability, information is subjective: if we already know something, being told it again provides no extra information. Furthermore, a new message may contradict a previous one. For instance, a friend calls to say he's just seen

(a)

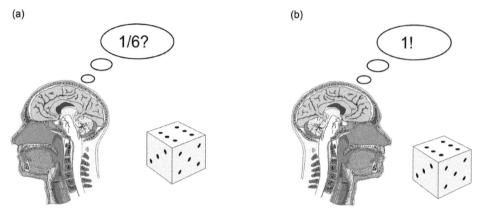

(b)

Figure 3.1 Subjective probability depends on past experience. A die has thrown a 6. But if you haven't looked at it (a), your probability of a 6 is 1/6. But when you do look at it (b), the new information makes the probability jump to 1.

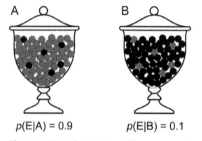

$p(E|A) = 0.9$ $p(E|B) = 0.1$

Figure 3.2 A chance setup. The two urns, A and B, each have 100 balls, each either red or black. But A contains only 10 black balls, whereas B has 90. Thus, the chance of drawing a red ball from A ($p(E|A)$ is 0.9, but for B ($p(E|B)$ it is only 0.1.

I've won the National Lottery – so for me U is about 25. If he calls again with the same message, U is unchanged. But if he calls to say that he got it wrong, and I hadn't won, U returns to zero. This point is discussed more fully in Appendix 1, Section App 1.7.3.

In the real world, information tends to be more nuanced than these binary messages asserting that one has or has not won the lottery. It is received as hints and cues that improve our stored model of how the world behaves or by deliberate sampling. As always, it is helpful to consider a tangible example. Suppose we have a pair of identical lottery urns, one (A) containing 10 black balls and 90 red, the other (B) containing 90 black balls and 10 red (Figure 3.2). Clearly, one is more likely to draw a red ball from A than from B. Formally, if we call E the event of drawing a red ball, we have a pair of conditional probabilities: $p(E|A) = 0.9$; $p(E|B) = 0.1$. Here the | sign means 'given', so we can translate $p(E|A) = 0.9$ as 'the chance of drawing a red ball from urn A is 0.9'. We are using 'chance' here to represent the probability of an event, derived from frequency or equipossibility, as opposed to 'probability', which is best reserved for subjective probability, in this case about which urn is which.

Now a friend challenges you to a game: while your back is turned, he tosses a coin to choose one of the urns, and withdraws a ball from it. Now you are shown the ball, which is red, and have to guess whether it came from urn A or urn B. This is a classic example in inverse probability. Rather than starting with a hypothesis (for instance, that this is urn A) and then calculating the chance of an event (for instance, drawing a red ball), we start with the event and have to calculate the probability of the hypothesis. Intuitively, it seems more likely the urn was B rather than A, but how much more likely? At this point, you have no reason to prefer one urn to the other, so we can call the probabilities of each of the urns having been chosen as $p(A)$ and $p(B)$, $p(A) = p(B) = 0.5$. Yet we feel differently about them. Can we express that feeling mathematically? The answer lies in a theorem that underlies virtually the whole of decision, Bayes' Law.

3.3 Bayes' Law

The Reverend Thomas Bayes (1701–1761) was a non-conformist clergyman who was also a mathematician, and in fact a Fellow of the Royal Society. The Law or Theorem that bears his name (Bayes 1763), published posthumously by a friend, was the first formulation of the mechanism, Bayes' Law, by which evidence leads to changes in probability.

The simplest derivation of Bayes' Law is to consider a pair of independent hypotheses A and B, and to ask how we calculate the probability of A and B both being true, in other words, estimating $p(A.B)$. Oddly enough, Bayes' own circumstances provide a good example: What is the probability of a given person being both (A) a Fellow of the Royal Society (FRS) and (B) a clergyman? One way to find out would be to get a complete list of FRSs, count them, and see what proportion that is of the population as a whole – giving us $p(A)$. Then we could see what proportion of those FRSs were also clergymen (Figure 3.3): this gives us $p(B|A)$, the conditional probability of B, given A. Then:

$$p(A.B) = p(A)p(B|A). \tag{3.1}$$

But we could equally have gone about it the other way round: starting with a list of clergymen (giving $p(B)$) and then finding out what proportion of them, $p(A|B)$, were also FRS. So:

$$p(A.B) = p(B)p(A|B). \tag{3.2}$$

From these two equations it is clear that $p(A)\, p(B|A) = p(B)\, p(A|B)$, and by rearrangement we then have Bayes' theorem:

$$p(B|A) = p(B)p(A|B)/p(A). \tag{3.3}$$

Why is this relevant to decision-making? Suppose A is some piece of evidence, E, and B is some hypothesis, H. Then:

$$p(H|E) = p(H)p(E|H)/p(E). \tag{3.4}$$

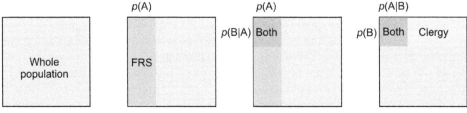

Figure 3.3 Of the whole population, a proportion $p(A)$ are Fellows of the Royal Society, and a proportion $p(B)$ are clergymen. So, the proportion of the population who are both is $p(B|A)$, which is also $p(A|B)$.

(Here, $p(E|H)$ is called the *likelihood* (Edwards 1972, 1974): it is simply the conditional probability of E given the hypothesis H.)

So Bayes' Law says that the posterior probability of the hypothesis, after receiving the evidence, is given by the prior probability multiplied by the likelihood, and divided by the probability $p(E)$ of getting the evidence at all. In practice we are nearly always comparing two or more hypotheses with the same event E, so it is convenient to use Bayes' Law in the form of *odds* (Appendix 1, App 1.7.4), the ratio between a pair of probabilities. So, for two alternative hypotheses A and B we then have:

$$\frac{p(A|E)}{p(B|E)} = \frac{p(A)}{p(B)} \cdot \frac{p(E|A)}{p(E|B)} \tag{3.5}$$

The term on the left is called the *posterior odds*, the next term is the *prior odds*, and the ratio of the conditional probabilities is called the *likelihood ratio*. So, the posterior odds are given by the prior odds multiplied by the likelihood ratio (this has the desirable consequence that $p(E)$ – in practice a difficult term to estimate – cancels out).

Returning to our game, the prior odds were 1, since $p(A)$ initially $= p(B)$. We already know that $p(E|A)$ is 0.9 and $p(E|B)$ is 0.1, so the likelihood ratio is 9; therefore, the posterior odds are $1 \times 9 = 9$. In other words, knowing the ball is red means it is exactly nine times more likely that A was the urn chosen, rather than B.

It is convenient to use equation 5 in logarithmic form, so that the multiplication becomes an addition. We can then say that:

log posterior odds = log prior odds + log likelihood ratio.

The log likelihood ratio or LLR comes up all the time in the statistical analysis of observed data, as it summarises how the data change our belief in different hypotheses. The LLR – also known as the *support* for hypothesis A against B afforded by E (Jeffreys 1936) – is in effect a measure of the relevant information that the evidence has provided (Edwards 1972). As we shall see, hypotheses and events have a kind of reciprocal relationship to each other: hypotheses predict the frequency of events, events establish the probability of hypotheses.

3.3.1 The Dominance of Priors

A crucial point here is that evidence modifies our beliefs, but cannot specify them: whatever we observe, the post odds are simply proportional to our prior odds, and this can sometimes give rise to errors of judgement. The final degree of belief depends not just on the evidence, but also on the initial prior probabilities. If a hypothesis is intrinsically very unlikely, it will take much more support before the odds reach an acceptable level than if it is rather probable. Two examples may make this clearer.

You have a coin that you suspect may be double-headed. You toss it, and it does indeed come down heads: clearly your suspicion is to some degree strengthened. More specifically, since the likelihood ratio is 1/0.5, the odds of it being double-headed are increased by a factor of two. You repeat the tossing, and in 10 consecutive tosses the coin comes down heads every time. So how certain are you that it is indeed double-headed? The total likelihood ratio over all trials is now 2^{10}, which is about 1000. Is it fair to say that the odds of it being double-headed are 1000:1? If we actually tossed a coin and got 10 heads in a row, would we really conclude that it was double-headed? No, we wouldn't, because our prior odds are not 1; the actual prior probability that a penny chosen at random is double-headed is surely much less than 50%. Even if as many as one in a million coins in general circulation was double-headed, we would still doubt it. The final odds would still be 1000:1 in favour of the coin being normal, and we would need to see 20 heads in a row before accepting an even bet on it being double-headed.

This problem arises all the time in medical diagnoses. The next example is very surprising, and shows just how important prior probabilities are. Suppose a certain disease has an incidence of 1% in the general population. There is a clinical test for it, which is pretty reliable: 90% accurate (that is, if you have the disease, there is a 90% chance of it giving a positive result; if you haven't, there is a 10% chance of it falsely indicating that you have the disease). Someone comes into your surgery, and you administer the test: it comes out positive. What is the probability that they have the disease? Intuitively, given the good reliability of the test, one might well think that they do indeed have the disease. If H_1 is the hypothesis that they have it, and H_2 that they haven't, then the likelihood ratio is 9. But the prior odds are only 1:99 and the post odds are 1/11. So, in fact it is overwhelmingly likely (11:1) that they do *not* have the disease!

3.4 LATER as a Bayesian Decision Device

The LLR is in effect a measure of the relevant information that the evidence has provided (Edwards 1972). In real life – especially in science – we may go on gathering evidence. Every time we do so, the old posterior odds become the new prior odds, and a little more is added on by the new evidence that comes from repeating the experiment. If your friend offers to repeat the draw (having returned the original red ball) and once again it is red, the new posterior odds are 9 × 9, or 81 – so it is overwhelmingly likely that A was the chosen urn. On a logarithmic scale, each successful repeat of the experiment raises the log odds by the same amount, equal to the LLR.

How might a Bayesian mechanism of this kind be implemented in the brain? Stripped to its essentials, we might imagine a neuron or group of neurons whose activity reflects the log odds favouring one of a pair of opposed hypotheses (for instance, that the visual field was moving to the left rather than to the right; or that a target is on the right rather than on the left). Initially, this decision signal S is at a level S_0, corresponding to the prior log odds. Then when information starts to arrive, for instance, from sensory stimuli providing evidence for or against the hypotheses, S will start to rise at a rate r reflecting the LLR of the evidence. Eventually it will reach a criterion level S_T, corresponding to odds so overwhelming that action is justified: the response is then initiated (Figure 3.4) (Noorani 2014). So supportive evidence from a stimulus arriving at a

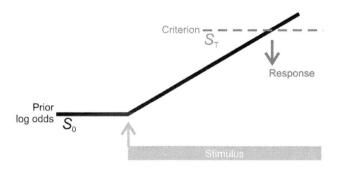

Figure 3.4 LATER as a Bayesian decision-maker. A decision signal, representing log odds, starts at a level S_0 (the prior log odds). In response to the stimulus, it starts to rise at a constant rate until it reaches the criterion level S_T, when it initiates a response. From Noorani and Carpenter (2016).

constant rate will tend to cause the log probability to rise linearly, eventually reaching a probability level (analogous to a significance level in statistics) which compels a response.

Does all this seem familiar? It is of course almost exactly what had previously been deduced from something apparently entirely unrelated, the distribution of reaction times (Schall 2003, 2005). Almost exactly, but not completely exactly: what is different – and not at all Bayesian – is the random variability itself. To understand how this randomness arises, and why it might be beneficial, we need more information about the underlying neurophysiology; for this reason, this important topic has to be deferred to Chapter 5. That apart, LATER – originally developed simply as an explanation for reaction times – turns out also to represent a kind of ideal decision-maker. In many ways, this is a remarkable conclusion. It provides an exact link between two concepts – reaction time and decision – that are at first sight completely unrelated. It is like building a bridge, and finding (with relief) that the two halves do finally meet up.

3.5 Behavioural Tests of LATER

Several aspects of the linear rise-to-threshold model are in principle susceptible to experimental falsification. LATER has the virtue of being unusually vulnerable, in the Popperian sense (Popper 1959). One fundamental point concerns the difference in the way its behaviour changes in response to the variation of different kinds of experimental variable: *stimulus* variables and *circumstantial* variables. Stimulus variables are those that depend entirely on the stimulus and cannot be manifest before the neural effects of the stimulus itself. They include such factors as intensity, contrast, size, position, and so on. Circumstantial variables are those whose value is determined before the start of a trial, and typically (though not necessarily) vary only slightly or slowly during a run. They include expectation, motivation, prior instructions, and arousal insofar as this is not influenced by a stimulus within its own trial. Of the parameters that characterise the rise-to-threshold mechanism, it is clear that changes in circumstantial variables will in general alter S_0 or S_T, and hence θ, and thus cause changes in the latency distribution corresponding to swivelling around the infinite intercept.

3.5.1 Expectation

The claim that LATER, a model originally derived empirically from the study of reaction time, is an embodiment of an 'ideal' decision-maker is a bold one, and correspondingly vulnerable to experimental testing. We can try to verify this functional interpretation by challenging its three main elements. For instance, a crucial test of LATER is to change the subject's expectation, which should cause S_0 to alter. In this way, provided the training period is long enough, one may set the subject's prior odds for a pair of targets to any specified level.

In a conventional step task, a trial starts with a central fixation target that suddenly jumps randomly with equal probability to left or right. To alter a subject's expectation, all we have to do is arrange for it to jump more often in one direction than the other (La Berge and Tweedy 1964). The latency in the more probable direction gradually reduces, and gets longer in the other direction, settling down after 50 or so trials.

LATER's prediction is then quantitatively precise: the decrease in latency to the more expected target and the increase for the less expected will be in direct proportion to the log prior probability for each target. Furthermore, the corresponding changes in latency

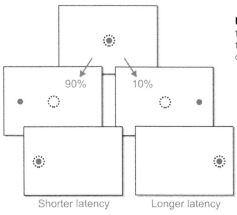

Figure 3.5 A prior probability task: in this case, the target is 10 times more likely to move in one direction than the other, leading to the development of a difference in latency in the two directions.

90%   10%

Shorter latency   Longer latency

(a)   (b)

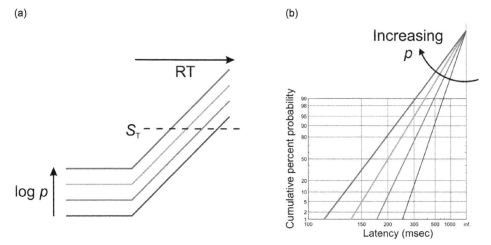

Figure 3.6 How altering prior probability in LATER should affect latency distributions. (a) Reaction time (RT) is linearly related to log prior probability, the starting point of the rise-to-threshold process. (b) Increased prior probability, p, causes the distribution to swivel around the intercept, reducing reaction times. From Noorani and Carpenter (2016).

distribution will take the form of changes in slope while k remains constant, so that the probit line swivels around its intercept (Figure 3.6). This experiment was undertaken in 1995 (Carpenter and Williams 1995), with full quantitative verification of both predictions (Figure 3.7): the rate of rise to threshold was equivalent to some 77 ms per log unit. A complicating factor is the increasing numbers of early responses as target probability increases, though their distributions also appear to swivel around the infinite intercept at $p = 50\%$.

Another way of altering the prior probability is simply to have a larger or smaller number N of alternative targets. Assuming equipossibility, the prior probability for any one target is $1/(N + 1)$ – the extra 1 is because one must also take account of the absence of the target – so that the median reaction time is given by $K \log(N + 1)$ (Hick's Law (Hick 1952)) where K is around 1.2–1.4.

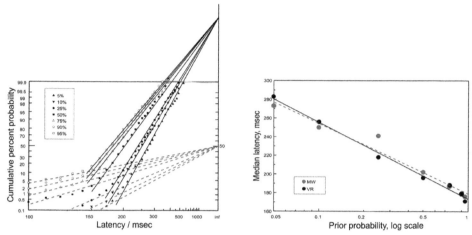

Figure 3.7 Observed effect of expectation on saccadic latency distributions. Raising S_0 reduces θ, resulting in swivelling of the reciprobit plot around the infinite intercept. (a) Reciprobit plot of saccadic latencies for one subject in trials for which the probability of a target appearing was varied as shown, exhibiting the expected changes in median latency, with a constant intercept. A similar effect occurs with the early responses (red asymptotes). (b) Linear relation between median latency and log probability in this task, for two subjects. Redrawn from Carpenter and Williams (1995).

Finally, an interesting question is how spatially localised these changes in expectation are. Do they affect prior probability over a wide area, or are they sharply confined to the position of the conditioning target? Along the horizontal axis, at least, the 'acuity' is surprisingly low: an isolated high-probability location reduces latency essentially uniformly over the whole hemi-field, with the opposite hemi-field unaffected (Adams, Wood et al. 2000). Having a high-probability locus in both hemi-fields has no effect at all.

3.5.2 Urgency

The next challenge to LATER is to check the prediction that alterations in S_T should also cause the distribution to swivel about its intercept.

We can alter a subject's sense of urgency simply by suitable instructions: either to respond as quickly as possible, and not to worry if errors are made, or alternatively to be as careful as possible, and take as much time as needed. To investigate urgency, it is helpful to use a difficult task, where errors are liable to be made, and a good choice is a modified version of Shadlen and Newsome's *random-dot kinetogram* (Shadlen and Newsome 1996, Reddi and Carpenter 2000). It consists of a large number of dots in continual motion: some move steadily in one direction, to left or right; the others move randomly. Instructions about urgency then have dramatic effects of the latency distribution: the main part swivels about a fixed intercept (as expected in LATER if the effect is to alter the criterion level). As with expectation, reduction in latency is associated with a large increase in the number of early responses.

Again, the prediction would be of a change in slope with constant k (Figure 3.8). However, we cannot be quite as precisely quantitative in our predictions as when we change prior probability, because although we may encourage the subject to be more or

(a)

(b)

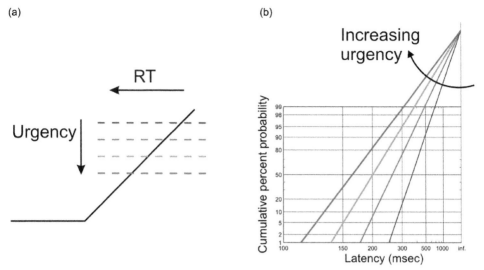

Figure 3.8 How altering urgency should affect latency distributions in LATER. (a) By lowering the threshold level S_T for initiating an action, increased urgency will result in a shorter reaction time. (b) As with increased prior probability, the result will be a swivelling of the distribution around the intercept, with consequent reduction in latency. RT, reaction time.

less careless or whatever, what we cannot do – as we can with expectation – is to specify a numerical value for the degree to which S_T ought to be affected. On the other hand, if one accepts the model, one could turn this around by pointing out that measurements of latency distributions would then provide a way of expressing degrees of arousal, or the effects of instruction, in a quantitative way with relatively little effort. So different degrees of urgency can in principle be calibrated against different prior probabilities, providing a numerical scale for urgency.

Figure 3.9 shows reciprobit plots of saccadic reaction times in an RDK task where the subject was told either to be slow and careful, or to respond as quickly as possible and not to worry about making mistakes. The distributions for careful and careless are strikingly different. The main distribution swivels about a fixed intercept, with an increased median latency when being careful. When careless, there is a huge number of early saccades.

3.5.3 Information Supply

Random-dot kinetograms (RDK) also provide a convenient way of manipulating the amount of *information* made available to the subject. If the proportion of dots that are moving coherently is high, the rate of information supply is greater. This should alter the mean rate of rise of the decision signal, and this in turn should cause the distributions to be shifted horizontally in a parallel fashion rather than swivelling, and this is indeed what is observed (Reddi, Asrress et al. 2003), Figures 3.10 and 3.11. It would be good to extend this line of investigation to other, more general examples where the rate of supplying information can be systematically altered. An obvious approach would be to alter signal-to-noise levels in the low-level sensory input (for instance, by reducing contrast), but as we shall see (Section 4.6.2), this appears to have its effect on a preliminary, detection stage that is distinct from the decision process implemented by LATER.

(a) (b)

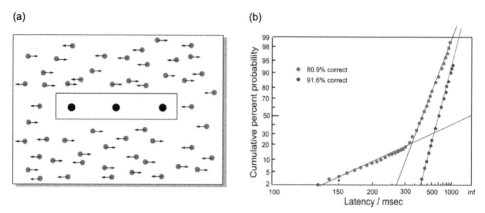

Figure 3.9 Effect on latency distributions of altering urgency. (a) The task: while fixating the central dot, the subject must estimate whether in the random-dot kinetogram (RDK; blue dots) the movement is mostly left or mostly right, and make a corresponding saccade to the left or right dot target. (b) Reciprobit plot of reaction times from one subject in this experiment, with instructions either to be as careful and accurate (blue) or as fast as possible, not worrying about mistakes (red). Note that high urgency generates a very large number of early responses. From Reddi and Carpenter (2000), Genest, Hammond et al. (2016).

(a) (b)

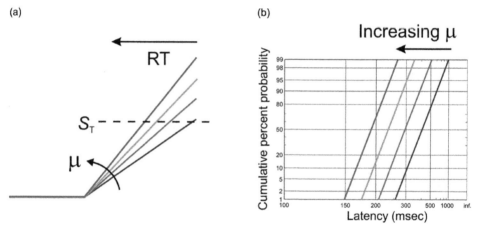

Figure 3.10 How altering the information supply should affect latency distributions in LATER. (a) Increased supply of information will increase μ, the mean rate of rise of the decision signal, resulting in a shorter reaction time (RT). (b) The result should be a self-parallel leftward shift of the distribution, with a consequent reduction in latency.

3.6 The Benefits of Procrastination

Be slow to resolve, but quick in performance.
John Dryden, The Hind and the Panther (1687)

Like any other biological responses, saccades are subject to evolutionary pressure. Contemplating the procrastination so vividly seen in Figure 1.5, Chapter 1, where we have to wait some 170 ms before generating a movement whose duration is only 30 ms or so, must lead one to ask what compensating advantage there is in a response that on the face of it is so obviously undesirable.

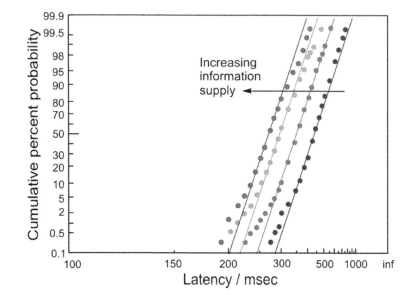

Figure 3.11 Observed effect on latency distributions of altering information supply in an RDK task. From Reddi, Asrress et al. (2003).

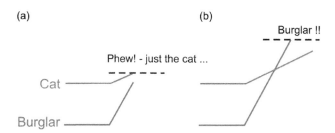

Figure 3.12 The cat and the burglar. If the criterion level for initiating a response is too low (a), too much weight is attached to the prior probabilities rather than actual incoming evidence (b).

The answer lies in a rather fundamental question: in general, how much weight do we attach to our existing expectations and internal models of the outside world – built up by Bayes-like mechanisms over a long period – compared with *new* information? Our internal models embody a lifetime of experience, but of course at any moment the circumstances may change. It is for this reason that playing the financial markets by strict application of Bayes' Law has not been a notable success (Smith, Dickhaut et al. 2002, Glimcher and Rusticini 2004). Crashes and booms can be triggered by events – a war, a change of US President – that have not been experienced before and therefore cannot contribute to the existing model.

Imagine you are alone at home, in bed, and hear a noise downstairs. What can it be? It might be the cat – in fact, it probably is. But it might be a burglar. The prior probability of cat rather than burglar is so high (Figure 3.12) that it is tempting just to go back to sleep again. But the sounds continue, and – ominously – they sound more burglar-like than cat-like – was that a match being struck? The probability of the burglar steadily overtakes that of the cat, and finally there is no escaping the necessity for firm action – so you pull the blankets over your head and pretend to be asleep.

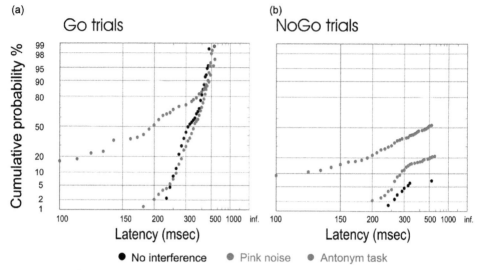

Figure 3.13 Effect of cognitive distraction (Halliday and Carpenter 2010). (a) Go trials under the three conditions (no interference, pink noise, antonym task), showing the marked increase in early responses as a result of performing the antonym task. The number of trials was 150 for *N*, and 300 each for pink noise and antonyms. (b) NoGo trials: the distributions are therefore for the latencies of error responses, and their asymptotes reflect the overall error rates for the three conditions. Error rates are greatly increased by the antonym task and are mostly due to early responses.

This example also highlights a question that often causes puzzlement: why have such a high criterion level? Surely for fast responses we ought to have as low a threshold as possible? But speed is not everything, and deliberate delay has the advantage of allowing more time to correct an impending response in the light of later-arriving information (Thompson, Hanes et al. 1996). Similarly, without procrastination, there may be too much weighting of the existing model in relation to the information actually being taken in. With it, we can make a judicious balance between previous experience and new knowledge: the longer the procrastination, the more we favour immediate information. So, in general we can favour the status quo rather than what may after all be an erroneous first impression: the political parallel (conservative versus radical) is obvious.

We can demonstrate this quite effectively by combining a difficult choice task – for example, where the subject is required to make a saccade to red targets and not to green – while simultaneously carrying out a completely different, and demanding, verbal one (Halliday and Carpenter 2010). In this particular experiment we were trying to show that the danger with using mobile phones while driving is not so much a physical matter of carrying out two actions at the same time, but rather that having a phone conversation imposes too much 'cognitive overload', generating responses that are indeed very fast but likely to be wrong (Figure 3.13). As a control, we presented meaningless 'pink' noise, which had little effect either on the incidence of early responses or on error rates. The result is that the usual descending tonic inhibition that partially suppresses more primitive responses from the superior colliculus is weakened, revealing its over-fast and erroneous responses.

Complex Decisions
Multiple LATER Units

When I 'choose' a book from the bookcase do I react fundamentally as does my microscopic acquaintance, amoeba, confronted by two or more particles, when it takes one of them? . . . From my fancy's plurality of possibles there emerges my de facto singleness of act. It leaves me with the impression of a decision.
Sir Charles Sherrington, Man on his Nature *(1940)*

In the real world, it is very rare for a single target suddenly to pop into view. In general, there are many potential stimuli that compete for our attention, and the decision to select one of them is the result of competitive interactions between multiple LATER units (Mackay, Cerf et al. 2012, Tatler, Brockmole et al. 2017). But before we deal with this kind of *spatial* complexity, we need to consider a particular aspect of *temporal* complexity. How do targets interact when presented sequentially rather than simultaneously?

4.1 Altering Prior Probability

We saw in the last chapter that prior probability has a profound effect on reaction time. When a target is more likely to appear on the left rather than the right, the latency for leftward saccades decreases and that for rightward saccades increases. This is an example of what might be called *static* prior probability, the result of a relatively long-lasting alteration in the initial level of the decision signal, S_0. It is reasonable to ask about the dynamics of this process: how quickly can S_0 alter to changed circumstances? There are really two ways in which we can try to drive S_0 up or down. We can suddenly change the prior probability of the stimulus being on the left or the right. Alternatively, we can use conditional probability, presenting in advance of each trial a predictive cue which the subject comes to associate with an increased probability of a particular target.

If in the middle of a step task experiment the prior probability of the target being on the left or right is suddenly changed – without telling the subject – unless the change is large the subject is normally unaware of the difference. Nevertheless, the latencies on each side gradually alter (Anderson and Carpenter 2004, 2006), until they reach the values they would have attained had the current probabilities been static. It typically takes some 70 trials to reach this final equilibrium. From a strict Bayesian point of view, every trial should summate equally with other trials. But the results from this experiment suggest a different conclusion: that there is a process of *forgetting*, such that the results of older trials are weighted less heavily than newer ones, being discounted by a Lethean factor λ (so the weighting is $(1 - \lambda)$. Typical values for λ are around 0.05. Since λ is effectively a measure of the speed of forgetting, it would make sense for it to be smaller in circumstances where the world is relatively stable and unchanging, but larger when things are more unsettled. It turns out that the whole process can be modelled at the neuronal level by a very simple quasi-Hebbian mechanism that modifies synaptic strength (see Appendix 1, App 1.9.1).

4.2 Cuing Tasks

In a cuing task, at some point during the foreperiod we present a cue that provides information to the subject about where, or when, the target is about to appear (Figure 4.1). This information may be totally reliable, so that the cue is an infallible indicator of what is about to happen, or – more usefully – it may be probabilistic, so that there is a relationship of conditional probability between the cue and the target (Fecteau and Munoz 2007). The cue may provide information about target location or about the time of its appearance. Since the cue itself must be sensed and recognised, it is likely to be more effective in modifying behaviour if there is a longer time between the appearance of the cue and of the target itself. In general, we would like to know the dynamics of this process, in effect the time-course with which S_0 changes after the cue have been presented. Partly because of the large number of types of cuing task that could be investigated, rather less work has been done on the time-course of cuing in general than one would like. Up to a point, the longer the time-interval d between the cue and the target, the larger the effect on latency, suggesting that the cue initiates a relatively gradual movement of S_0 with a time-course of around 200 ms (Figure 4.1). In one study (Ware, Blount et al. 2001), targets were normally presented at $d = 300$ ms after the cue, but on a few trials at other times. The smaller that d is, the smaller the effect on latency; more precisely, S_0 itself builds up exponentially from its initial value to one representing the conditional probability associated with the cue. In addition, the stronger that the predictive power of the cue is – the larger the value of the conditional probability – the larger the effect on S_0.

There are many other tasks in which the cuing effect is present, but sometimes not very obvious. For instance, in an ordinary step task, the offset of the fixation spot could be regarded as a kind of cue in the sense that it is followed by the appearance of one of the targets. This effect is even more marked if there is a delay between the offset of the fixation target and the subsequent target appearance (the gap task). However, discussion

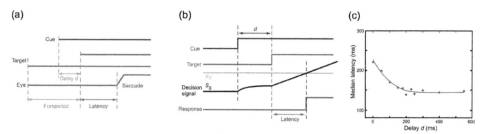

Figure 4.1 A cuing task. (a) The protocol: at the end of the foreperiod, a cue is presented that provides information about the location or timing of the subsequent target, which appears after a delay d. (b) The cue initiates a process that causes S_0 to change, so that the rise-to-threshold begins at a different level. (c) Probing the cuing process. Here the target was normally presented 300 ms after the cue, but on occasional trials it appeared earlier or later. The graph shows, for one subject, how latency falls as the delay d increases, reflecting the time-course of S_0: the line is an exponential function. Replotted from Ware, Blount et al. (2001).

of this commonly used protocol must be postponed to Section 4.5.2 as it also involves a phenomenon yet to be fully discussed, lateral inhibition.

4.2.1 Foreperiod as Cue

Just as prior information about the location of the target reduces latency, so does prior information about when it is likely to appear. So, in designing experimental protocols, it is important to ensure that this is as far as possible unpredictable. For instance, if the foreperiod is the same on every trial, latencies fall dramatically. Often, the experimenter arranges for the foreperiod to vary simply by specifying a range of values with an upper limit, and then choosing one specific value at random, with equal probability over the whole range. It is also necessary to have a fixed component as well to avoid a foreperiod of zero. However, in one respect this is not ideal, since during the foreperiod the expectation that the foreperiod is about to end will get larger and larger as it approaches the upper limit. This can be seen in Figure 4.2, where the reciprobits for different foreperiods show the swivel round the intercept characteristic of changing the prior probability. An alternative to this *ageing foreperiod* is to abolish the upper limit, and instead arrange things so that the probability of the foreperiod ending is constant at any moment – a non-ageing foreperiod. So whereas with an ageing foreperiod the latency alters as a function of the foreperiod for any particular trial, with a *non-ageing foreperiod* latency is on average the same whatever the value of the foreperiod (Oswal, Ogden et al. 2007). The conclusion is clear: we should use non-ageing foreperiods (unfortunately, in practice not many experimenters do!).

4.2.2 Sequences

Another way of increasing the prior probability of a target is when there is a repetitive sequence, for instance, 'left, left, right, left'. Because of the predictability, latencies are then gradually reduced. However, if we disrupt the sequence – for instance, by one cycle of 'left, right, right, left' – the latency for the unexpected target is increased, and it may take several recurrences of the original sequence for the system to get back to normal (Anderson, Yadav et al. 2008, Anderson and Carpenter 2010).

4.2.3 Task-Switching

Sequences clearly have to be learnt, implying an initial period during which the system is in effect being programmed. The same sort of thing occurs in task-switching. An

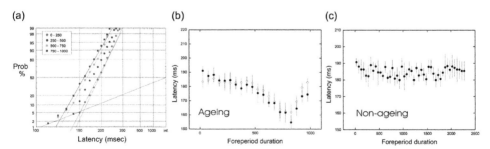

Figure 4.2 (a) Reciprobit plots comparing four different foreperiods; (b) latency as a function of foreperiod with an ageing protocol; (c) with a non-ageing protocol (Oswal, Ogden et al. 2007).

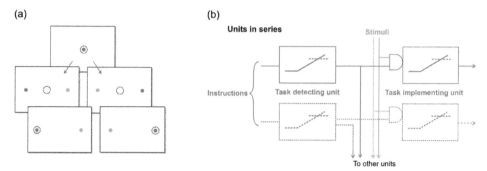

Figure 4.3 Task-switching. (a) The colour of an instructional target (in this case, red) tells the subject what colour of target to look at in a choice task. (b) Two stages are then required, in series. The first, task-detecting, unit determines what task is required, and selects the appropriate second, task-implementing, unit.

example is a pair of targets of different colours – say, red and blue – being presented on each trial, and the subject is instructed that throughout the run to make a saccade to blue targets and not to red. Here the programming is in effect the result of a verbal instruction and remains in force throughout a run; this is an example of a Go / NoGo task (see Section 4.3).

Alternatively, instead of verbal instruction, we could indicate to the subject that blue is the target to look at simply by presenting a blue target at the fixation spot before the run (Figure 4.3(a)). This then opens the possibility of doing the experiment dynamically rather than statically by presenting either red or blue instructions before some of the trials during the run itself, which remain in force until a different instructional colour is presented. This task-switching protocol implies two decision units (Figure 4.3(b)). One must register the instructional target, and the other must identify the targets themselves. All this turns out to be relatively easy to model accurately, with the instructional decision unit simply selecting one or other of the two possible programs (Sinha, Brown et al. 2006). The latency for switch trials is much larger than for the intervening controls, around 180 ms or so, as would be expected if we have in effect two LATER units in series. The same conclusion follows from the fact that if a longer period is allowed after the instruction to switch, before presenting the pair of targets, the extra latency for switch trials is reduced, eventually to zero.

4.3 Races and Choices

A simple binary choice task (Figure 4.4) is easy to implement using LATER. What we need are two LATER units corresponding to the two possible responses that race against one another. The one that reaches the finishing line first determines which of the two possible responses is actually made. If the support for one is much higher than for the other, then it will be chosen practically all the time. The distributions for correct and incorrect responses can be calculated relatively easily (Appendix 1, App 1.8.2).

Earlier, we looked at Bayes' Law, and saw that by working in terms of odds, the ratio of the probabilities of two hypotheses, we avoid the difficulty of having to calculate $p(E)$, the underlying probability of the event E occurring irrespective of any particular hypothesis. However, in the real world hypotheses do not normally come in pairs: typically, there will be several rival hypotheses, and a given piece of evidence will support

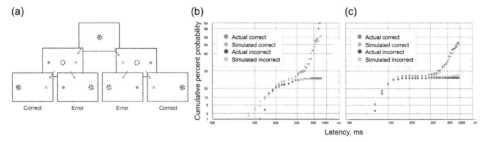

Figure 4.4 (a) Choice task (Go / NoGo), in which the subject has been instructed to look at the red target but not the green. In practice, errors are sometimes made, especially when the targets are similar to each other. (b and c) Two examples of the resultant distributions for correct and incorrect responses (Noorani, Gao et al. 2011). Note that these are 'incomplete' distributions, showing percentages of the total number of trials, rather than only trials with the same outcome.

some of them more than others. In search tasks, for example, the thing we are looking for may be at any of a large number of different locations within the visual scene.

One solution is to do exhaustive pair-wise comparisons of the different possibilities – H_1 versus H_2, H_1 versus H_3, H_2 versus H_3, and so on – but this rapidly leads to a very large number of decision units being needed. Furthermore, a second stage of computation will be required to translate the activation of one particular unit into a final choice of action. If the H_1-versus-H_2 unit reaches its threshold, is that sufficient reason in itself to choose H_1, without considering also how H_1 has fared against all the other hypotheses?

Another solution is not to attempt to calculate probabilities or odds at all. If all we want to do is make a choice of the best-supported hypothesis, we really do not care what the absolute degree of support is for each one. Provided the scale-factor is the same for all, a relative measure will do perfectly well. So all we need is a set of decision units, one for each hypothesis, that calculates a logarithmic version of equation 4, with the log $p(E)$ term (which would otherwise be subtracted from each) simply omitted:

$$S = \log p(H) + \log p(E|H).$$

With information arriving continuously, S will again rise (or fall) steadily, starting at $S_0 = \log p(H)$, the log prior probability, and rising with a mean rate $\mu = \log p(E|H)$. To make the best choice, all we need do is run a race between the units for all the hypotheses (Figure 4.5). These different possibilities are discussed further in Appendix 1, App 1.7.7.

In other words, if all we want to know is which hypothesis is most probable, and don't care *how* probable it is, a simple race between a set of LATER units provides an economical mechanism for making the choice. We do also need a mechanism by which the winner stops the others in their tracks, so that only a single response is made. This means some kind of lateral inhibition: a topic discussed in Section 4.4.

The simplest choice is when there are just two alternatives. For instance, a subject may be presented with a red target on one side and a green one on the other, having previously been instructed always to look at the red target. In this situation, they are liable to make mistakes, performing a perfectly good saccade to the incorrect target (Figure 4.6). This is in fact exactly what LATER would predict. To some extent, the incorrect LATER unit will also receive some support from the sheer existence of the target; the correct target is additionally supported by whatever the attribute is – colour, in this case – that should be determining the choice. So, both units will be activated to

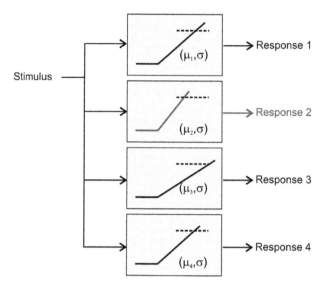

Figure 4.5 Races between LATER units. Four units driven by the same stimulus, with different rates of rise; the winner (red) is the one with the fastest rise, that is, 'first past the post'.

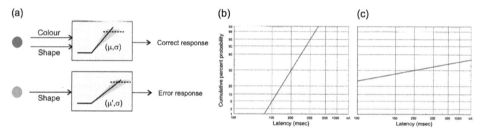

Figure 4.6 How errors arise with LATER. (a) Errors of commission: the subject is instructed to look only at red targets, but both units are activated to some extent by the mere existence of the target. Because of the variability of the rate of rise of the decision signal, on some trials the subject will therefore look at the wrong target. (b) The intercept *k* is so large that all trials will reach completion. (c) But if it is smaller (in this case, equivalent to 70%), then a substantial number of trials will generate no response (errors of omission).

some extent, with the correct one having a larger value of μ than the incorrect one. Because of the random rate of rise, this means that occasionally the incorrect unit may happen to win, generating an error response (Noorani, Gao et al. 2011) (Figure 4.6). If the critical attribute is not very clearly different between the two targets – if, for instance, the two colours are very similar – then more will be made than when they are clearly distinguishable, because the two values of μ will be close to each other. This might be called an error of *commission*, but LATER is perfectly capable of making errors of *omission* as well. If the rate of rise μ is small, then the intercept *k* will be small as well. Since it represents the probability of not making a response at all, this makes it likely that LATER will simply fail to respond to the original stimulus (Figure 4.6(b)).

What can we then predict about the latency distributions? Conventional reciprobit plots of correct and error responses are not very informative in this situation (Figure 4.7 (a)). What is much more useful is to plot *incomplete distributions*. These are cumulatives of responses as a percentage not of each individual count but of the total, with errors and

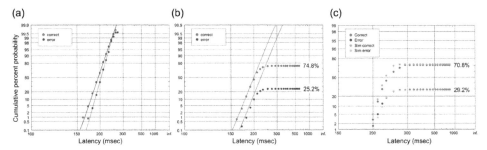

Figure 4.7 Plotting competitive reaction times. (a) Conventional plot in which the cumulatives for each case (red, correct; blue, error) are percentages of each individual total. (b) An incomplete plot, in which the cumulatives are shown as a percentage of the total number of trials, errors plus correct responses. As a result, they flatten off at a level corresponding to the percentage of correct and error responses (in this case, 74.8% and 25.2%); the lines represent the expected distributions for each LATER unit considered separately; simulated data, $N = 1000$; $\mu = 5.0$, $\mu' = 4.5$, $\sigma = 0.5$. (c) Data from an actual experiment using two targets of quite similar colour, together with the results of a simulation as in (b), with the values $\mu = 4.44$, $\mu' = 4.16$, $\sigma = 0.35$. $N = 400$ for the observed and simulated data.

correct responses combined (Figure 4.7(b)). The resultant curves have a characteristic shape, rising linearly, but then flattening off at a level that represents the overall percentage of each kind of response. (The mathematics behind this is explained in Appendix 1, App 1.2). Figure 4.7(c) shows some actual data of this kind, from a task in which a subject had to saccade to the slightly redder of two, very similar pink spots, making nearly 30% errors. By running a simulation of the two competing units we can get the underlying values of mean rates of rise, μ and μ', which one might then hope to relate to the physical degree of similarity of the targets. We have to run a simulation to do this, because as soon as we have more complex models than just a single LATER unit, the interactions between the components means that even in conventional, complete, plots such as Figure 4.7(a) we cannot expect to get recinormal distributions and thus straight lines.

4.4 Lateral Inhibition

A complicating factor is an almost universal property of neural networks in the brain, lateral inhibition. Its function is to exaggerate the differences between the activities of neighbouring units, both in sensory and motor systems, leading to better discrimination and the elimination of aspects of the signals that are common to all the units, such as uniform backgrounds or noise (Mach 1875, Mach 1886). They are most easily seen in the visual system. In the set of graded stripes in Figure 4.8(a), for instance, one has the impression that in each stripe the side next to the brighter neighbour is not as bright as the other side. This is because the brighter stripe is laterally inhibiting the corresponding neurons. Lateral inhibition has been demonstrated in the saccadic system, not just in behaviour (Munoz and Istvan 1998, Ludwig, Gilchrist et al. 2005) but also in the interactions between individual competing neurons (Figure 4.9), for instance, neurons in the frontal eye fields that seem to be involved in the selection of saccadic targets (Schall and Hanes 1993) (see Section 5.1.4) and also between the centre and peripheral areas of the superior colliculus (Munoz and Wurtz 1993a, 1993b, 1993c).

(a)

(b)

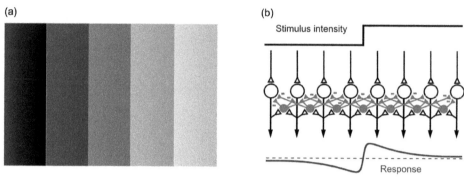

Figure 4.8 Lateral inhibition. (a) A set of graded grey stripes. At each boundary one has the illusion that the stripe is darker in the region near a lighter stripe, and lighter near a darker stripe. (b) Schematic representation of one kind of neural network giving rise to lateral inhibition. Via inhibitory interneurons (blue), each neuron in the layer inhibits its neighbours over a certain distance, leading to enhancement of any differences in their activities and an exaggerated spatial pattern of activity.

(a)

(b)

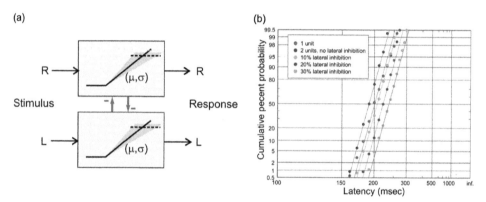

Figure 4.9 The effect of lateral inhibition during a race. (a) Two racing LATER units, as in Figure 4.7, but with mutual feedback lateral inhibition. (b) Simulated distributions for a single target and for two simultaneously presented targets, the subject having a free choice, together with different amounts of lateral inhibition as shown. The effect of the inhibition is to increase latency, shifting the curves to the right ($N = 1000$).

4.5 Asynchronous Tasks

So far, we have examined a variety of tasks in which we present the target just once in each trial, though it may be preceded by a cue of some kind. Now we need to consider a number of situations in which there is more than one target, which may be presented asynchronously, in other words, at different times during the trial.

4.5.1 Precedence

One of the clearest examples of an asynchronous task is the *precedence* task (Leach and Carpenter 2001). Here a central target jumps either to the left or to the right as before, but on some trials the other target also comes on, after a short delay d. We tell the subject to look at whichever one they like. Provided such trials are interleaved with ordinary one-target trials randomly to the left and right, most subjects choose each side with

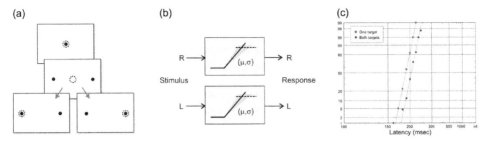

Figure 4.10 Free choice with two simultaneous targets. (a) The protocol: the targets are presented simultaneously on left and right, and the subject makes a saccade either to one or the other, at will. (b) This situation can be modelled by two LATER units activated simultaneously in parallel. Sometimes one will reach threshold first, sometimes the other. The expectation is that the average reaction time will be less than for either target on its own. (c) Some actual data from a subject responding to a single target in a step task, and to two presented on each side simultaneously. The responses in the latter case are slower rather than faster, and can be modelled with about 15% lateral inhibition (N = 200) (Leach and Carpenter 2001).

roughly equal probability. If d is long, then the subject always saccades to the target that appeared first; but as it is reduced, the choice of targets becomes stochastic. There is a tendency to choose the target that came on first, but sometimes it is the other that is chosen. The smaller d is, the greater the probability of choosing the second target, until $d = 0$, when each is chosen with equal probability.

We can model this in LATER as a race between two identical units, the first past the post determining what response is made (Figure 4.10). One thing this immediately demonstrates is that the randomness in the two competing units must be *independent*; otherwise ,the first to appear would always 'win'. Another feature of the behaviour is at first sight difficult to explain. In any race, one would expect that on average the reaction time would be less than for just one target on its own, since we are selecting for the faster of the two responses. But this is not at all what is actually seen (Figure 4.11(c)): the entire distribution is shifted to the right relative to the one for a single target: in other words, the average response is *slower*, not faster. How can this be? If we add lateral inhibition of this kind to a pair of LATER units that are racing against each other (Figure 4.10(a)), the result is rather as if each runner in an actual race were devoting part of their energy to elbowing their rival in the ribs or trying to trip them up. This means that the overall time for the race is longer on average than if they were running separately. In Figure 4.10, the simulated distributions shift to the right as the degree of lateral inhibition is increased. (Here percentage of lateral inhibition means what proportion of the output of one unit is subtracted from that of the other). The actual data shown in Figure 4.10 can be modelled in this way with a value for the lateral inhibition of about 15% (Leach and Carpenter 2001). The instructions to the subject turn out to be very important: if told to look at whichever target comes on first, most subjects cannot perform the task, or at least only for very large values of d: they tend to agonise long after the targets have been presented, trying to make up their mind about which was first. But if the instructions are simply to look at whichever target happens to catch their attention, with no mention of the fact that one comes on before the other, then most (but not all) subjects perform very consistently. As in most saccadic experiments, it's better for the subject not to think too much (Appendix 3, App 3.4.3).

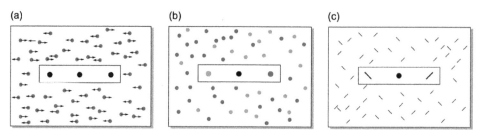

Figure 4.11 Distributed counting tasks. (a) Random-dot kinetogram (RDK) or random-dot tachistogram (RDT); (b) colours; (c) orientations. In each case, the subject initially fixates the central black dot, and then makes a saccade to one of the two targets on each side that signifies their judgement of the stimulus that is in the majority.

4.5.2 Gap and Overlap

In the classic gap task (Figure 4.11(c)), instead of the peripheral target appearing at the same time as extinction of the fixation point, there is a short delay or gap. This results in a reduced latency, and often a greater incidence of early and express responses. In some ways, this is an unsatisfactory task, as the existence of the gap has two separate effects. The first is that the offset of the fixation target acts as a cue, increasing the expectation of the peripheral target and would therefore be expected to reduce the latency. The second is to do with the lateral inhibition mentioned above, which creates a mutual antagonism between stimuli currently being fixated and new ones appearing in the periphery. As a result of the absence of the fixation target during the gap, there will be relative enhancement of the response to the peripheral target, which is likely to reduce the latency still further. Fortunately, it is not difficult to disentangle these two effects by presenting an explicit cue at the time when the fixation target would otherwise have disappeared (Story and Carpenter 2009).

4.6 Global Evaluation of Extended Stimuli

So far, we have considered tasks in which relatively small targets are presented at well-defined positions and times. This is not a situation that often occurs in the real world, where we are normally faced with an extended background that may be static or moving, and eye movements can be made to any part of it. These may be for the purpose of searching for a particular target, or the instructions may simply be to scan the scene spontaneously with no particular goal, acquiring general information about what is displayed. In the laboratory, but seldom in real life, we can also ask a subject to make judgements about aspects of the background – for instance, whether it is predominantly red or predominantly green – which can then be reported by making a saccade to one location rather than another.

4.6.1 Judgements Based on the Scene as a Whole

An artificial but extremely informative experiment is to present a subject with an extended field containing a number of items, for example red and green dots, and ask them to indicate which kind of item is in the majority by making a saccade to one of two targets on the left or right. These are in effect distributed counting tasks, but the subject is told not literally to count them, but form an impression of the answer while holding the gaze on the central fixation target. Commonly used attributes include colour, movement to left or right, or orientation (Figure 4.11). The stimulus may consist either of two distinct populations of one uniform population mixed up with a second population that is random. In a random-dot kinetogram (RDK), for instance, a typical stimulus would consist of a proportion a of the total set of N dots moving together in one direction, with the others executing a random walk (a Type 1 counting task), whereas for colour a proportion a of dots might be red and the remaining $(N - a)$ green a Type 2 counting task). The mathematics underlying these kinds of discrimination are presented in Appendix 1, App 1.9. Clearly, for a Type 2 task, the closer a is to $N/2$ the more difficult the discrimination will be, whereas a Type 1 task is more like detecting contrast, with the difficulty increasing as a is reduced.

Finally, a refinement of RDK is to make the movement of the dots instantaneous rather than continuous, a random-dot tachistogram (RDT) task (Genest, Hammond et al. 2016). This has the advantage of removing an irrelevant source of extra noise, and means that after the jump no information can be obtained from the final appearance of the field, so that there is a well-defined and extremely short period of time when information is actually received. An additional practical advantage is that each trial can then be much shorter.

4.6.2 Two Stages of Judgement: Detection and Decision

So far, we have presented the case for regarding LATER as an ideal Bayesian decision-maker. However, there is one aspect of it that at first sight does not look at all ideal: the random variability embodied in σ. Where does it come from?

Of course, all biological systems are subject to the unpredictable disturbances technically known as *noise*. The importance of the signal-to-noise ratio in sensory systems is well understood (Fatt and Katz 1950, Barlow 1957, Green and Swets 1966, St-Cyr 1973), and its influence can be estimated quite accurately through suitable psychophysical tasks such as measuring thresholds. Consequently, it is natural to suppose – as in most early studies of reaction time, and as implied by some modern ones – that the unpredictable variation in reaction time is simply a reflection of the sensory noise that is present at the input. In such a scheme, the signal and noise are integrated to generate a rising signal that is superficially similar to that in LATER, but instead of being linear it obeys random walk statistics.

However, several kinds of evidence strongly suggest that under most conditions, sensory noise does not contribute significantly to the variability of reaction time. The signal-to-noise ratio of the kinds of targets commonly used to evoke saccades is very high, with contrasts at least a log unit above threshold, and this component is negligible (Schall and Bichot 1998). But as the contrast is reduced to levels near threshold, latencies dramatically increase (Carpenter, Reddi et al. 2009) (Figure 4.13). The relationship between contrast and detection time is very close to what would be expected if the average rate of rise of the detection signal were a logarithmic function of contrast, as is found, for instance, at higher levels of the visual system (Campbell and Kulikowski 1972), using human, visually evoked potentials. Changes in the stimulus can only affect the rate of rise, μ, and possibly its variance, σ^2; however, in this case the conclusion must be modified by the existence of a prior, random-walk, stage of stimulus *detection*. So, at high contrasts, reaction times are dominated by a LATER-like *decision* mechanism, but

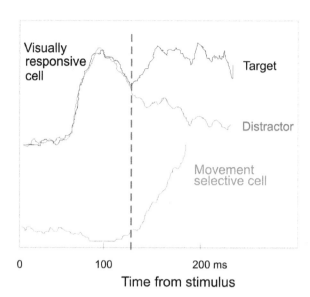

Figure 4.12 Recordings from stimulus-related (red and black) and movement-related (blue) neurons during a distractor task. At first, neurons whose receptive fields contain a distractor rather than a target follow essentially identical time-courses, until colour information arrives (dotted line) when they diverge. If the stimuli are high contrast, the time of this divergence varies very little, and is too small to explain the overall variation in reaction time. The rise-to-threshold of movement-related neurons then begins, and variability in their rates of rise correlates with overall reaction time. Modified, after Schall and Bichot (1998).

when targets arc less visible, it is the detection stage that dominates, so that the overall behaviour is more like a random walk (that is, random small ups and downs along a trajectory). It is for this reason that there has in the past been some conflict between these two descriptions of reaction time behaviour (Carpenter and Reddi 2001, Ratcliff, Carpenter et al. 2001).

So, as we reduce target contrast, eventually we start to see an added component of reaction time due to the time taken to detect the target against its noisy background. This has been thoroughly confirmed by recordings from neurons in frontal cortex (Schall, Hanes et al. 1995, Schall and Bichot 1998, Schall and Thompson 1999). Figure 4.12 shows superimposed recordings from individual stimulus-related cells in frontal cortex in a colour distractor task, in which a saccade must be made to a target that is a different colour from the others. Because information about colour arrives relatively late, at first the activity in neurons whose receptive field has a distractor is identical with those that don't. Then when colour information finally arrives, the activity of the disappointed distractor cell declines and for the others remains high. Under high-contrast conditions, the moment at which this divergence starts varies very little, certainly not enough to cause the overall variability in the saccadic latency, and it coincides with the start of the rise-to-threshold for movement-related cells.

The conclusion is clear: there is not just a single stage of rise-to-threshold, but instead two in series. Clearly, the detection of elements of a stimulus against a noisy background is a component of what has to be done in order to make a decision for action (Barlow 1980), Figure 4.13; but except in the case of the simplest, hard-wired reflexes, there must be at least one more stage, in which the separate pieces of information about the existence of individual fragments of the stimulus are put together to see whether together they provide evidence for the existence of the object in the outside world to which the subject has been instructed to respond, Figure 4.14.

That the decision part can introduce an extra time in addition to what is needed for detection is evident from anti-saccade tasks (see Section 4.9.4), where a subject instructed

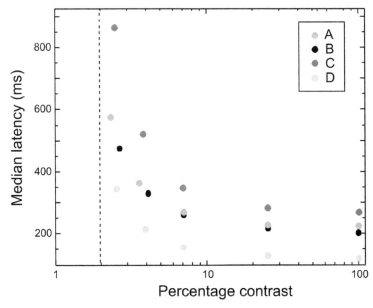

Figure 4.13 Median latency for single targets as a function of their contrast, in four subjects. At high-contrast levels (right), contrast has little effect; but as contrast is reduced to near threshold, the latency rises sharply. From Carpenter, Reddi et al. (2009).

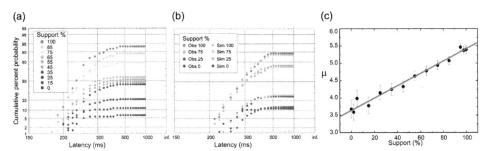

Figure 4.14 Effect of altering support (i.e., percentage of dots moving in the same direction) in an RDT task as in Figure 4.11(a). (a) Set of distributions for one subject. (b) Observed and simulated distributions for another subject. (c) Best linear fit (red line) of μ to data from another subject. Modified from Genest, Hammond et al. (2016).

to look in the opposite direction to a target does so with much longer latencies, though the stimuli are identical (Hallett and Adams 1980). Although the need for a model that separates the detection and decision components of reaction time has sometimes been explicitly recognised (Ejima and Ohtani 1987), it is not easy to formulate or test quantitatively without using the extra information that is provided by full latency distributions rather than simply means or medians. What is proposed here is a detection stage of random-walk type, followed by a decision stage with a linear rise-to-threshold (Figure 4.16). On the simple assumption that mean rate of rise in the random walk is linearly related to log contrast, such a model makes a good job of predicting the general characteristics of the distributions of latencies, and their error rates, as well as their medians (Figure 4.15).

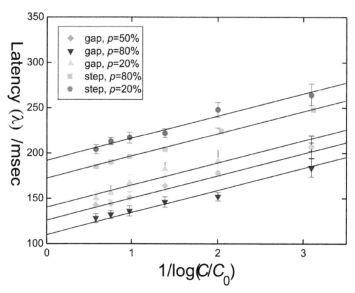

Figure 4.15 Saccadic latency as a function of reciprocal log contrast in a human subject for different tasks (gap or step) at different prior probabilities (Carpenter, 2004).

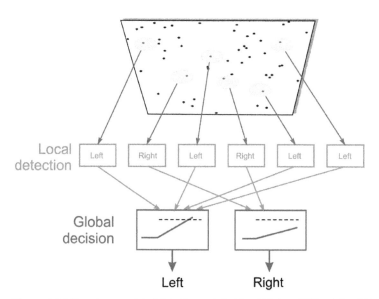

Figure 4.16 Two-stage model of detection and decision. This is an RDK task, in which the subject must judge whether the predominant direction of motion is to the left or right. In the first, detection, stage, individual neurons (green) with limited receptive fields (blue) signal whether the motion of any dots that they see is in their preferred direction. This information is then pooled and sent to corresponding LATER units (red), which race against each other to determine the final response.

The idea of two stages in series – detection and decision – has quite a nice parallel with the operation of a court of law. Here there is a sharp distinction between the witnesses and documents that are examined to establish the truth of individual items of fact (Lindley 2000), and the decision by the jury as to whether all these facts amount to a

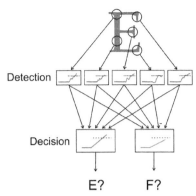

Detection

Decision

E?   F?

Figure 4.17 In general, discrimination must necessarily be a two-stage process. The first stage consists of the detection of fragments of evidence concerning the existence of particular features. The second stage consists of deciding whether this set of fragments supports one hypothesis (in this case, 'E' rather than 'F') better than others.

sufficiently strong case against the accused (Reddi 2001). In the same way, the first stage in recognising a letter 'E' is the detection of a multitude of individual features – lines, edges, and corners – by essentially independent, specialised, neurons at a relatively early stage in the visual system (Figure 4.17). Then all this evidence must be assembled in order to make the decision as to whether this is in fact an 'E' and not 'F' or 'H'. Different kinds of factors will affect the two stages. Low-level attributes such as brightness and contrast will influence detection; prior probability and urgency will influence the final decision, just as evidence as to character or past convictions may sway the jury. However, there is another aspect of the court of law that has an important parallel in the overall decision process, which has not so far been mentioned. The court's job is not just to attempt to discover truth; it must also pass sentence. In doing so, it must consider, in part, what are the likely benefits or drawbacks of one course of action rather than another.

Although this quasi-Bayesian process represents a good procedure for arriving at truth, it does not tell us what to *do* about it. However faultlessly I can prove to you that if you touch an overhead power cable, you will be killed, I cannot prove to you that you should not touch it. The possible role of the *utility* of different outcomes in choosing one course of action rather than another – perhaps even ignoring which is actually more likely to be true – is discussed in Section 6.4.

In this two-stage model, neurons in the first stage integrate stimulus information over time until a trigger criterion is reached: at this point they 'raise their hands', continuing to fire to indicate that they have detected a target, until the end of the trial. Thus, the signals it sends to the second stage are taken to be all-or-nothing binary signals that simply indicate that some potential stimulus has been detected. The persistency of these signals, held constant until the decision is complete, is clear from the fact that very brief stimuli generate the same prolonged decision time as targets that are longer in duration (Section 4.7.1). In addition, the 'hand-raising' behaviour has been demonstrated in neurons in the middle temporal region (Smith, Zahn et al. 2001).

The function of the second, or decision, stage is to choose between competing hypotheses concerning the existence of complete objects in the outside world, using as evidence the information about localised individual stimulus elements provided by the first stage. Because it is presented with constant binary signals that look certain (though they may not in fact be so; we feel a confident certainty about noise-ridden decisions (Barlow 1990)), the rise-to-threshold is not a random walk but linear, its purpose a procrastinating and thus integrative one. The decision stage is the one that is influenced by prior probabilities, by the number of alternatives, by urgency, and no doubt by the utilities associated with various outcomes.

4.7 Stimulus Factors

4.7.1 Duration

Finally, there is the effect of curtailing the duration of the stimulus. If there were actually integration of the sensory stimulus over the time span of the rise-to-threshold, then one would certainly expect curtailment of the target's appearance to have a drastic effect, since the decision signal would not then reach the threshold and no response at all would be made (Figure 4.18). While behaviour of this kind is certainly seen on the simple assumption that mean rate of rise in the random walk is linearly related to log contrast (Bloch's Law, Figure 4.19) for durations of 50 ms or less with easily visible targets (Bloch 1885, Hildreth 1973, Tolhurst 1975), the prediction if rise-to-threshold represented actual integration of stimulus information would be that Bloch's Law should extend to the whole duration of the reaction time. In fact, experiments in our laboratory on saccadic reaction times have shown that in a situation where median latencies are around

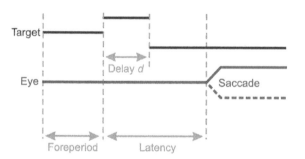

Figure 4.18 A step task with curtailed stimulus. The trial begins in the conventional way, but after a duration *d* the target disappears: there may or may not be a saccadic response.

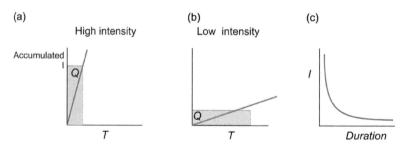

Figure 4.19 (a and b) Schematic representation of Bloch's Law: the threshold is determined by the total quantity of light received (the time-integral of the intensity). So, at high intensities this threshold is reached earlier than at low intensities. (c) This means that threshold is essentially a reciprocal function of stimulus duration.

200 ms, curtailment of the target's appearance has essentially no effect on the form of the distribution until the duration is reduced to less than about a quarter of the total expected rise-to-threshold time.

4.7.2 Contrast

An important factor that affects one's reaction time to a visual stimulus is the contrast of that stimulus. In order to understand how changes in contrast of a stimulus affect reaction times, experiments were performed where the contrast of a visual stimulus was changed whilst subjects were expected to make saccadic or manual responses to the stimulus. It was found that reaction times to increments in contrast could be explained by a separate stimulus 'detection' stage occurring prior to a 'decision' stage; this detection stage was portrayed as a rise-to-threshold model as well whose rate is determined by the change in log contrast of the stimulus, whereas the rise-to-threshold decision stage that subsequently occurs is not affected by the stimulus contrast (Taylor, Carpenter et al. 2006).

4.7.3 Why a Linear Rise?

The natural interpretation of any rise-to-threshold model in the context of target detection is in terms of a sequential statistical test for significance, in which the accumulation of information is paralleled by the rise of some decision variable to a threshold representing a criterion for acceptance of a hypothesis (S_T behaving very like a conventional significance level). It is well established that there is no more efficient way of proceeding, provided that the significance indicator is scaled in such a way as to be equivalent to a sequential probability ratio test (which amounts to accumulating log likelihood) (Wald 1947, Wald and Wolfowitz 1948, Green and Swets 1966). The applicability of this approach to models of reaction time seems first to have been realised by Stone (1960), and has subsequently formed the basis of many other studies (La Berge 1962, Grice 1968, Laming 1968, 1973, Pacut 1977, Vickers 1979, Watson 1979, Pacut 1980, Smith 1980). It was also consonant with rather earlier ideas derived from information theory: other things being equal, reaction time should be proportional to the quantity of information required to reach a decision with a specified probability of being correct, a notion that had been most clearly confirmed by experiments in which the number of possible responses, and thus prior probability, was systematically varied (Hick 1952, Hyman 1953, Gregory 1956, Welford 1959).

However, there are two essential respects in which this general class of model – sequential testing – is quite distinct from the linear rise-to-threshold proposed here. In the first place, a process equivalent to an optimal sequential probability test must have independence of consecutive samples, which means that the trajectory of the resultant rise-to-threshold will not be linear, but instead have the form of a random walk (that is, a series of noisy ups and downs as the trajectory gradually rises). Second, although the effects of manipulation of the prior odds seems in general to accord with the ideas of information-limited reaction time, the effects of altering the signal-to-noise ratios of the targets themselves do not. For comfortably visible targets, altering the contrast has considerably less influence on reaction time than would be expected if detection were the limiting factor, though as threshold is approached the effects on latency become disproportionately large. Figure 4.14 illustrates this clearly, with a greater difference in median latency as a target is reduced from 8% to 6% than from 100% to 12%. As we have seen, the implication is that the detection of the stimulus elements that constitute the target is a separate stage of processing that precedes the decision about whether the target as a whole is present or not. Both stages accumulate information and therefore perform integration. But whereas the detection stage integrates a signal with continually varying noise added to it, generating a random walk, the second stage – integrating the relatively static signals generated by the output of the first stage – is therefore linear.

4.8 Scanning and Searching

What we have been talking about nearly exclusively have been evoked movements, triggered, for instance, by the sudden appearance of a visual stimulus. But in the real world rather than the laboratory, objects seldom suddenly pop into view. More commonly, we are faced with a relatively static scene, yet we still make saccades – perhaps two or three every second. Can the occurrence and timing of these spontaneous movements also be explained by LATER?

In one sense, such saccades are in fact evoked. The sudden appearance of a new, displaced, retinal image at the end of the preceding saccade is in itself a powerful stimulus that would be expected to trigger the next movement. Thus, the time between the end of one saccade and the beginning of the next, the intersaccadic interval or ISI, can be regarded as a kind of latency (Van Loon, Hooge et al. 2002, van den Berg and van Loon 2005, Roos, Calandrini et al. 2008). Indeed, when plotted as reciprobits, ISIs show many of the characteristics of ordinary evoked latencies. As can be seen in Figure 4.20, their distributions are qualitatively similar to evoked ones, but differ in two respects: the median latency is typically longer, and there is usually a prominent early population. Another complication is that the very first saccade made in the sequence generally has a different latency distribution than the second or subsequent ones (Beintema, van Loon et al. 2003, Mackay, Cerf et al. 2012, Tatler, Brockmole et al. 2017), presumably because it lacks the history that is an important determinant of the duration of the ISI. Figure 4.21 shows reciprobit plots of saccades made whilst viewing more natural scenes.

4.8.1 Reading Text

A particularly important and well-studied example of saccadic scanning of a static scene is reading. Compared with more general scanning or searching of 'natural' scenes, it is

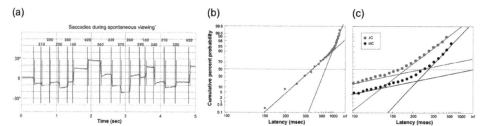

Figure 4.20 (a) A series of spontaneous saccades made while viewing a static display on a computer screen, with their intersaccadic intervals (Roos, Calandrini et al. 2008). (b) Reciprobit plot of intersaccadic intervals whilst carrying out a real-world task – making a cup of tea (Land, Mennie et al. 1999); (N = 401). (c) Two subjects carrying out a sequential visual search task: the distributions show the latencies of the second saccade made in each sequence. Replotted from van den Berg and van Loon (2005).

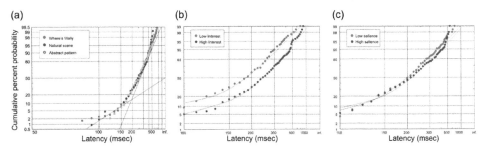

Figure 4.21 Spontaneous scanning of visual scenes. (a) Reciprobit plot of a subject making spontaneous saccades to three very different kinds of image: a 'Where's Wally' picture (Handford 1987), a natural scene, and a regular, abstract geometric pattern of checks (Roos, Calandrini et al. 2008). (b) A subject scanning static natural scenes on a computer monitor, showing the difference in distributions between targets of high and low 'interest' (i.e., how popular they are as targets of saccades). (c) The same data set, but this time divided into high and low visual salience; the difference is not statistically significant (Tatler, Brockmole et al. 2017).

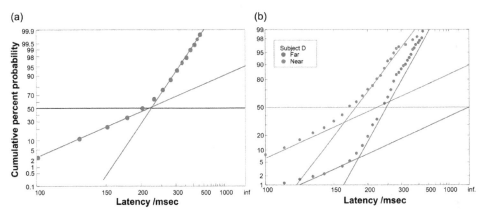

Figure 4.22 Reading. (a) Intersaccadic intervals while reading, with prominent multi-unit early saccades (Rayner and Pollatsek 2012) (N = 1000). (b) Subject making saccades while reading, to words that are near or far from current fixation (Carpenter and McDonald 2006).

subject to a number of intrinsic constraints. For most languages, the saccades are essentially horizontal, forming a series of steps that typically begin at a roughly constant horizontal position on the left (corresponding to the start of a line of text), and typically finish at a point on the right corresponding to the end of the line. In addition, reading the next line of text requires a vertical saccade, and – especially when the text is in some way challenging – there may be *regressions*, in which a backwards saccade is made to some point within the area that has already been scanned. Figure 4.22 shows a reciprobit plot of intersaccadic intervals while reading (McDonald, Carpenter et al. 2005); other authors (Rayner and Pollatsek 1989, Epelboim, Booth et al. 1994) have published conventional ISI histograms for reading that show similar characteristics when replotted in reciprobit form. Finally, to gather information from the text, the size of each step must be regulated to correspond with the size of the letters and the difficulty of assimilating the information that is presented. As Javal noted in his pioneering study of eye movements while reading (Javal 1879), the size of saccades is roughly scaled to match different distances or different sizes of font. As far as regulating the size of the steps is concerned, there are really two extreme possibilities.

The first, and more obvious, is simply to continue to fixate at a given location until the information available there has been fully extracted and then to move on to the next locus (Just and Carpenter 1980). This is likely to result in the most thorough interpretation of the meaning of the text, but at the cost of an unnecessarily long intersaccadic interval, since any decision about where to look next must follow completion of the process of comprehension. That decisions are in fact being made that are influenced by what is seen by the parafovea, and its meaning, is shown by the fact that saccades are more likely to land on the words themselves, and are influenced by expectation, including the context (and therefore the meaning of the next word to be processed) (Rayner and Fischer 1996).

An alternative strategy is to pay no attention to the underlying meaning at all, the eyes then scanning the text at an average rate matched to the difficulty of the content. When this average rate is too high, errors of comprehension arise that trigger a regression, and also a lengthening of the underlying ISI (O'Regan 1984). An analogy:

> Trucks deliver pea-pods to the Acme Pea Factory, where Chuck feeds them into a hopper that delivers them to an automated assembly line that extracts the peas from the pods and puts them into cans. All kinds of things can affect the rate of canning: the size of the pods, the proportion of defective peas, not to mention problems with the assembly line itself. Ideally, one should adjust the rate of putting pods in the hopper to match the rate the cans leave the line. But even if Chuck could see the cans coming out – he can't, because he's in a different room – it takes ten minutes for a pod put in at one end to emerge as peas in a can at the other, which is too long to take effective action. To allow for variation in the rate of processing, a warning light turns red when the hopper's getting too full, and green when it's getting too empty. Chuck's instructions are to slow down a bit when the light is red, and speed up when it's green.

In such a scheme, the oculomotor system is illiterate: the eyes walk through the text as our feet walk across a landscape, with equal indifference to the view.

The truth probably lies somewhere between these two extreme positions, and could perhaps be explained by a model that extends LATER by dealing more exactly with where saccades land rather than when they are initiated. Such a model has been proposed, the so-called LATEST (Linear Approach to Threshold Explaining Space and Time). The essence of the LATEST model is that it weighs up the relative likely benefit from remaining at the current fixation point or moving to a new target, and takes into account such factors as the size of the required saccade (see Figure 4.22(b)). (McDonald, Carpenter et al. 2005, Carpenter and McDonald 2006) It is fully discussed in Section 4.8.7.

4.8.2 Reading Music

Music reading shares many of the constraints associated with reading ordinary text, and imposes some extra ones of its own. In the first place, the vertical position of a note on the clefs conveys vital information, so that a substantial number of saccades are vertical rather than horizontal (Furneaux and Land 1999). On the other hand, even in sight-reading an experienced performer can use hints about the harmonic progression, and melodic clichés that enable them to predict aspects of the music that are not fully seen, and this kind of prediction is probably more marked than is the case for ordinary text. If

(a)   (b)   (c)

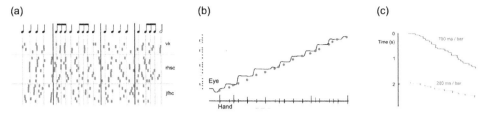

Figure 4.23 Reading music. (a) Three subjects reading the same line of music on different trials: there is often good consistency between trials, but not all fixations are on notes or bar-lines. (b) Recording of a single performance by one subject: the left-hand axis shows the music text; the two experimental traces (eye and hand) show the subject's responses; the red dots indicate when the subject tapped, in relation to what the text required. It can be seen that the eye is always slightly ahead of the performance itself, especially near the start. (c) Influence of performance speed on the pattern of eye movements. The subject is reading the same musical text at a fast tempo (above) and a slow one (below). It is obvious that many more fixations are made at the slower tempo and they tend to be shorter in duration. Modified from Carpenter and Kinsler (1995).

an actual performance is in progress, then there are time constraints; if the tempo is fast, the musical performance may be limited not so much by manual dexterity as by being unable to gather reliable information from the score sufficiently quickly (Figure 4.23(c)). The result is typically not a complete breakdown of the performance, but rather inaccuracies: a larger part must necessarily come from guessing on the basis of past experience rather than genuinely translating the notes into correct movements. These problems will be manifested in errors in the performance itself. The LATER parameters are altered to encourage guessing, lengthen the ISI, and lower the threshold (Figure 4.23(c)) (Carpenter and Kinsler 1995, Furneaux and Land 1999).

4.8.3 Optokinetic Nystagmus

Presented with an extended visual field full of individual elements all moving together with the same direction and velocity, the oculomotor system assumes that this must be because it is the *eye* that is moving, generating retinal slip. The retinal sip velocity is then used as an error signal, evoking a compensatory steady movement of the eye intended to match the velocity of the retinal slip – an example of a gaze-holding movement (see Section 1.1). However, the eye obviously cannot move forever in one direction, so this compensatory movement is interrupted at intervals by saccades in the opposite direction, tending to bring the gaze back to the centre. These two components together – slow phase and quick phase – are called optokinetic nystagmus (OKN, Figure 4.24(a)), a type of gaze-holding eye movement that evolved very early, and can be seen even in the most primitive organisms (Walls 1962, Carpenter 1992, Land 1995).

Figure 4.24 (b,c) shows measurements of the time-intervals between consecutive saccades during optokinetic nystagmus in different human subjects and with different speeds and directions (Carpenter 1993, 1994). They conform rather accurately to the standard pattern, again with a large proportion of early responses, which in all cases but one are a good fit to a recinormal distribution having $k = 0$.

4.8.4 Relation between Evoked and Spontaneous Saccades

All this suggests a common mechanism of decision-making for saccades evoked by sudden visual targets and for those made spontaneously in viewing static scenes,

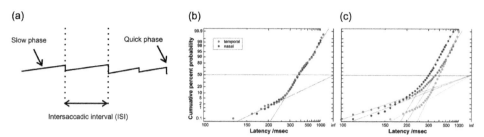

Figure 4.24. (a) Schematic drawing of optokinetic nystagmus (OKN). (b) Intervals between OKN quick phases for a single subject in the nasal and temporal directions: the distributions are statistically indistinguishable (K-S test; N = ca. 600 each). (c) OKN intervals in three subjects, with different stimulus speeds: both directions combined (N = ca. 1500 each) (Carpenter 1994).

applying to the timing of saccades in reading, in nystagmus, and in systematic visual search. In addition, very few studies have published raw histograms of ISIs for spontaneous saccades whilst carrying out everyday activities under 'natural' conditions (Land, Mennie et al. 1999), or in more controlled search tasks (van den Berg and van Loon 2005). They too show two segments of different slopes, a steeper main distribution with a long median, and a substantial population of early responses with a shallower slope (van Biervliet 1899).

4.8.5 The Origin of the Rightward Shift

Could this rightward shift in latency distributions be due to lateral inhibition? The visual stimulus revealed at the end of the preceding saccade consists of not just two but an entire visual field's worth of new competing targets, so one would expect any such mechanism of mutual lateral inhibition to be greatly accentuated. Saccadic latency is, for instance, increased by some 10 msec when the movement of the target coincides with a sudden contrast-reversal of a background grating (Crawford 1996), and the influence of shifting backgrounds that lie well outside the classical receptive field on the activity of visual neurons has been long established both in the retina (McIlwain 1966, Barlow, Derrington et al. 1977) and in the lateral geniculate nucleus (Fischer and Krüger 1974).

We can find out by comparing a target moving against a fixed background – as occurs in natural scanning saccades – with the target and background moving together as a whole (Figure 4.22(a)). In the first case, there is only one new target, so no competition: in the second case, all the elements suddenly appear in a new location, generating a great deal of competition. If this is the cause of the rightward shift in the latency distribution of spontaneous saccades, then a comparable shift should be seen under these artificial conditions. Against a stationary textured background, the distribution of latencies is very similar to what is found in a conventional step task with a uniform background, generating a single straight line on a reciprobit plot (Figure 4.25). But when the background moves with the target, the distribution shifts to the right by some 40 ms: being parallel implies that the difference is – as would be expected from lateral inhibition – due to a reduction in the mean rate of rise μ of the decision signal, rather than to changes in S_0 or S_T. In addition, the effect of the moving background is almost identical to what is seen with spontaneous movements (Roos, Calandrini et al. 2005).

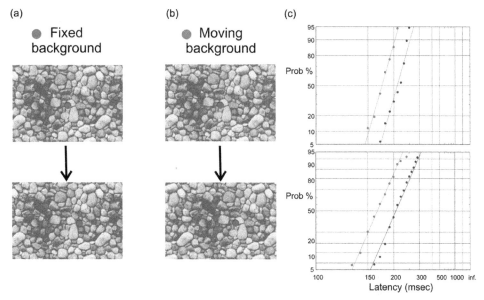

Figure 4.25 Comparison between a fixed and moving background. (a) The target moves but the background does not. (b) The target and background move equally. (c) A moving background (blue) slows the distribution, moving it rightward in a self-parallel fashion; this is characteristic of the effect of lateral inhibition (see Figure 4.11). Modified, after Roos, Calandrini et al. (2008).

4.8.6 The Increase in Early Responses

The other major difference between evoked and spontaneous saccades is that the latter show a greatly increased early population. Why might this be? One characteristic of early saccades is that they become much more frequent when stimuli are predictable. This is in keeping with the sense that the early population represents relatively automatic, reflexive responses, probably associated with a relatively low-level structure such as the superior colliculus, normally tonically inhibited by higher-level, probably cortical, decision mechanisms. A functional dichotomy of this kind seems first to have been proposed by Harris (Harris 1989), and an equivalent process of procrastination is an intrinsic feature of LATER (Carpenter 1981). A systematic study of altering the prior probability of saccadic step targets (Carpenter and Williams 1995) showed a systematic increase in the size of this population from 0.5% to 10% as the stimulus probability increased from 0.05 to 0.95, their distributions appearing to fall on a straight line swivelling about the origin k.

If we think of a spontaneous saccade as being, in effect, evoked by the preceding saccade and the new retinal image that it creates, then one important characteristic of this stimulus is that it is exceptionally easy to *predict*. We could scarcely have more information in advance about its timing (since we caused it!), and its amplitude and direction are similarly known almost perfectly before it happens. So, it would not be surprising for spontaneous saccades to display the increased proportion of aberrantly fast early saccades characteristic of highly predictable stimuli. To test this, we again arranged for the target to move randomly as described for the fixed background above. However, after a 250 ms delay, it returned to its original central position (Figure 4.26). Thus, the same target and background were presented first when timing and direction

(a)

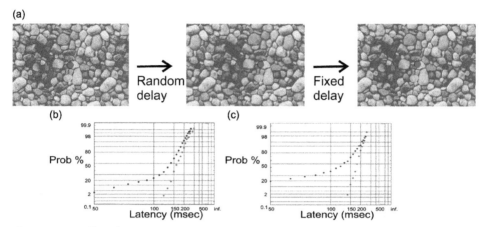

Figure 4.26 (a) Effect of extreme predictability on incidence of early response. The target and background moved together: (b) after a random delay from the start of the trial; (c) with a fixed delay and amplitude. As a result, the probability of an early saccade increased from about 3% to about 20%. Modified, after Roos, Calandrini et al. (2008).

were completely unpredictable, and then when they were completely certain. The resulting distributions were dramatically different: when the target was predictable, there was a large early component that was absent when it was unpredictable (Figure 4.26). When lateral inhibition and expectation were *both* increased, the simulation could fully account for the distribution of ISIs (Roos, Calandrini et al. 2005, figure 5B).

4.8.7 The LATEST Model

LATER is primarily a model of the timing of saccades: as a consequence, it can also predict choices between alternative targets. What it does *not* claim to do is predict the amplitude and direction metrics of the resultant saccade. However, it turns out that a small modification to LATER does in fact enable it to make quite a good job of predicting metrics in static scanning tasks, as well as timing and choice. This modified version is called LATEST (Tatler, Brockmole et al. 2017) (Linear Approach to Threshold Explaining Space and Time).

The concept underlying LATEST is that when scanning a static pattern, apart from interactions between possible targets, at a more fundamental level there is competition between the targets and the possibility of not moving at all: 'Go' versus 'Stay'. If there is still information to be extracted from the current fixation, that will favour 'Stay'. On the other hand, if a new potential target seems likely to provide more information, that will bias the decision favour of 'Go'. Competition of this kind seems first to have been suggested by Beintema, (Beintema, van Loon et al. 2003) with a choice between 'make saccade' and 'keep fixating'; by framing this concept within LATER, it is possible to generate quantitative predictions concerning saccadic amplitude and direction. As would be expected, the decision rate (i.e., μ) for the Stay unit is influenced by factors describing the current fixation and also the preceding saccade (Figure 4.27(a)), whereas for the Go unit it is determined by factors relating to the destination of the proposed saccade (for instance, 'semantics', the likely amount of information at that location), together with

(a)

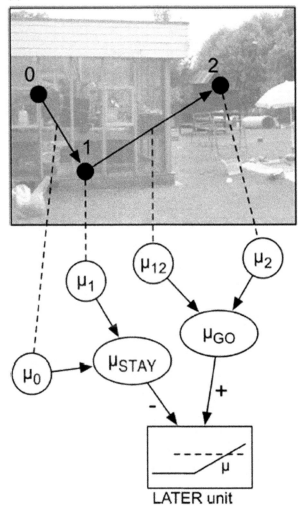

Figure 4.27 The LATEST model. (a) The overall μ for a given saccade (in this case, from fixation 1 to 2) can be regarded as the result of two competing processes: μ$_{Stay}$, representing the tendency to wish to remain at the current fixation in order to complete the processing of information, and μ$_{Go}$, the tendency to want to obtain new information from the next fixation. In addition, μ$_{Stay}$ is influenced by the preceding saccade, and μ$_{Go}$ by factors to do with the new saccade. (b) Examples of how the overall μ is influenced by these various aspects. Modified, after Tatler, Brockmole et al. (2017).

factors relating to the trajectory of the saccade about to be made, such as its direction and amplitude. As can be seen in Figure 4.27(b), 'semantics' works in opposite directions for Stay and Go. Increased information at the proposed location increases the decision rate, but reduces it at the current fixation. Taking all these factors together, it is then possible to make better predictions of both the temporal and spatial aspects of individual saccades.

(b)

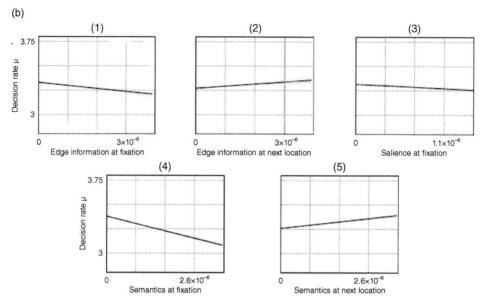

Figure 4.27 (*cont.*)

4.9 Stop Signals and Cancellation

So far, we have considered only situations where a target triggers the generation of a corresponding eye movement. But there are several situations in which the response to a target is suppression rather than generation of a response. They fall into two categories: extrinsic and intrinsic. *Extrinsic* means that the suppression is the result of prior instructions to the subject telling them to suppress a movement they would otherwise make; *intrinsic* implies a situation where the subject is given no particular instructions about suppressing a response, but where the logic of the protocol – for instance, a change in the ultimate destination of the saccade – means that the previously planned response is no longer appropriate.

In both cases, responses can be modelled with considerable precision by designating certain LATER units as 'Stop units', whose output inhibits or abolishes the 'Go units' that would otherwise generate an eye movement. Focused discussions on this topic are provided in reviews elsewhere (Carpenter and Noorani 2017, Noorani 2017, Noorani and Carpenter 2017), but here we discuss the salient points behind our understanding of stop mechanisms in the brain and how we study them experimentally.

4.9.1 Countermanding

The simplest and most thoroughly studied example of extrinsic suppression is the *countermanding task* (Logan and Cowan 1984, Hanes and Schall 1995, Patterson and Schall 1997, Hanes and Carpenter 1999, Asrress and Carpenter 2001, Ozyurt, Colonius et al. 2003, Walton and Gandhi 2006, Boucher, Palmieri et al. 2007, Emeric, Brown et al. 2007, Salinas and Stanford 2013, Schmidt, Leventhal et al. 2013). Here the subject is told that if a second target (the Stop signal) appears on some trials, they are required to

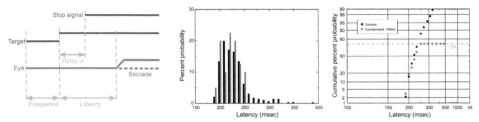

Figure 4.28 Countermanding task. (a) The protocol. It begins like a conventional step task, but on some trials a Stop signal appears after a delay *d* that instructs the subject to withhold the impending saccade. (b) Results from a countermanding experiment. Depending on *d*, countermanding may or may not be successful: the larger the *d*, the less likely that the saccade is withheld; the black bars are the control trials, the red are trials with Stop signals at 100 ms, only 28% of which resulted in successful cancellation. (c) The corresponding distribution of responses (unpublished data).

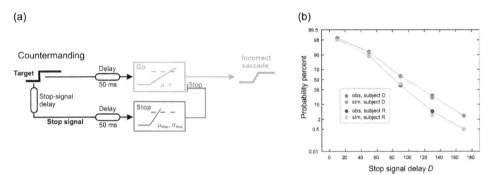

Figure 4.29 Modelling countermanding. (a) After the Stop-signal delay, the Stop unit is activated. If it reaches its criterion threshold before the Go unit, the movement is aborted. (b) Observed and simulated percentages of trials where the cancellation is successful, as a function of the Stop-signal delay. Modified from Hanes and Carpenter (1999).

withhold the movement that would otherwise have been made. The behaviour is stochastic, with the movement successfully cancelled on some trials but not others. The longer the period between presentation of the primary target and presentation of the Stop signal – the Stop-signal delay, *d* – the less likely it is that the movement will be successfully cancelled (Figure 4.28(c)). The behaviour can be modelled in terms of a race between 'Go' and 'Stop' processes (Hanes and Carpenter 1999, Boucher, Palmieri et al. 2007, Schall, Palmieri et al. 2017), Figure 4.29. An important difference with the precedence task (which is intrinsic rather than extrinsic) is that – perhaps because cancellation is a simpler operation than selecting a different target – the Stop process is more rapid than the Go, so that reliable cancellation can occur even with relatively large values of *d*.

4.9.2 Wheeless

In the Wheeless task (Wheeless, Boynton et al. 1966, Noorani and Carpenter 2015), which is special case of the double-step task (Becker and Jürgens 1975, Becker and Jürgens 1979, Camalier, Gotier et al. 2007), we present the subject with a series of trials of which some are simple step tasks and act as controls. But in the remaining experimental trials, after a delay *d* the target jumps to the alternative target position. The

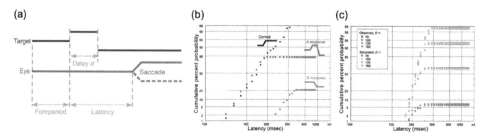

Figure 4.30 The Wheeless task. (a) The protocol begins like a step task, but in some trials (as shown here), after a delay *d*, the target steps across to the opposite side; sometimes the subsequent saccade is in the same direction as the original step (an A response), otherwise in the opposite direction (a B response). (b) Data from a single subject performing this task, with a delay *d* of 100 ms; at first the A responses follow the same distribution as in the controls, but then cease as the B responses begin to appear. (c) Observed and simulated data from one subject for four different values of *d*. Modified from Noorani and Carpenter (2015).

subject is not given any explicit instructions but simply told to follow the target. The behaviour is then stochastic: on some experimental trials, the subject saccades to the first target and then jumps to the second (an A response: see Figure 4.30), in the remainder they jump straight to the second (a B response), ignoring the original target. The larger the *d*, the more likely is an A response. Behaviour in this task can be modelled by LATER using a similar arrangement to the model for the Go / NoGo task, predicting latency distributions for all responses in this task remarkably well. In the model, an A response unit is triggered by the stimulus; after a delay *d*, the Stop unit is activated, which cancels the original A response if it has not already occurred; at the same time as triggering the Stop unit, the B unit is activated and rises toward threshold.

In many ways, this is a better task than countermanding (Noorani and Carpenter 2015). It saves time, since it generates data on every trial, whereas successful cancellation in countermanding means that there is nothing to measure. It also means that we do not have to give the subject prior instruction about what to do (and that the subject does not have to remember those instructions!), making it feel like a simpler task for a subject to perform.

4.9.3 Go / NoGo and Errors

Another situation that calls for an intrinsic Stop signal is the Go / NoGo task, where the subject is instructed before the run to make saccades to one class of target but not others. In this scenario, subjects often make saccades to the 'wrong' target, generating errors. For instance (Figure 4.31), they may be told to make a saccade to a green target (appearing on either side, the correct response) but not to red (the error). The reason why a Stop signal is needed in this case is that it takes longer for the brain (Schall and Hanes 1993, Thompson, Hanes et al. 1996, Thompson, Bichot et al. 1997) to respond to the colour of a target than to its existence and position (here we take this extra delay as 60 ms). In this way, there is a close analogy with the countermanding task, where colour information needs accounting for before a. correct response can be given with confidence. As a result, Go units will at first be activated on both sides, before the red unit is suppressed by a Stop signal originating from the colour of the red target. As a result of this intrinsic delay from colour information processing, mistakes will be made (some 40% in Figure 4.31(c)) if a decision is made by the brain before colour information arrives. A race-to-threshold

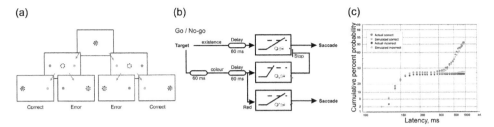

Figure 4.31 Go / NoGo task. (a) Protocol. After the foreperiod, a target appears either on the left or right, and may be red or green. The subject is instructed to make saccades to green targets but not red. (b) A model for this task, using two Go units (for red and green) and one Stop unit (for red). (c) Observed and simulated distributions for this task in one subject. Modified from Noorani, Gao et al. (2011).

model of this nature, with a Go unit triggered on appearance of a visual target followed by a Stop unit and another, more refined Go unit initiating when colour information is evaluated in the brain, accurately predicts the quite complex response time distribution from human subjects performing this task, emphasising the power of such a model in explaining behaviour (Noorani, Gao et al. 2011). In comparison with the Wheeless task where a response is generated in every trial, the Go / NoGo task has some inefficiency as an experimental system because a large proportion of trials (those with no responses, i.e., correctly stopping of saccades) do not contribute to the reaction time distributions.

It is an interesting notion that errors are made when the brain responds to a stimulus before all the necessary information arrives, and although this is exemplified well here in the Go / NoGo task with colour information, this is by no means the only situation in which this occurs. For example, we discussed earlier that when we are distracted, we tend to make more errors: an experiment with a Go / NoGo task where a subject had to make saccades to a specific colour but not others whilst simultaneously talking on a mobile phone (designed to distract them) led to many errors and also some responses that occurred much earlier than would otherwise occur if the subject had not been so distracted. Response time distributions in this scenario can be accurately recapitulated with incorporation of an 'early' Go LATER unit, suggesting that when extra cognitive loading distracts the cerebral cortex, then more primitive brain regions (likely the superior colliculus) can instead make saccadic decisions when they would otherwise be tonically inhibited by the higher cortical areas (Halliday and Carpenter 2010).

4.9.4 Antisaccades

Especially amongst clinicians, the *antisaccade* task is extremely popular, in some ways more than it merits (Hallett and Adams 1980). Here the subject is required to do something rather complex and *extremely* unnatural: when the target appears on the right, they are to make a saccade to the left, and when it is on the left, to the right (Figure 4.32). There may or may not be some kind of marker permanently visible to indicate more exactly where the saccade is meant to end up, but more commonly we don't mind very much how large the antisaccade is, only that it is in the 'right' (i.e., wrong) direction. As we shall see in Appendix 2, the reason for the clinical popularity of antisaccades is that they are difficult to execute without making mistakes. There is a powerful tendency to look at the target rather than away from it (a 'prosaccade'), so that the task requires a very strong and natural response to be inhibited, while generating

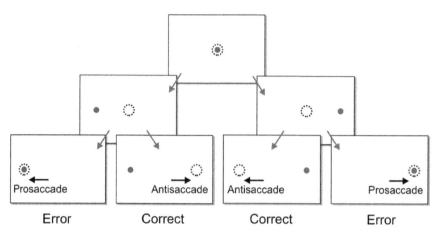

Figure 4.32 Antisaccade task. The protocol is as for a conventional step task, but the subject is instructed to make a saccade in the opposite direction to that of the target.

another response that is unnatural and slow because it is only slightly related to the stimulus and requires an additional stage of remapping to be performed. As a result, even 'normal' people make many mistakes, and a wide variety of clinical conditions of various kinds (Hutton, Joyce et al. 2002, Condy, Rivaud-Péchoux et al. 2004, Hutton and Ettinger 2006) cause significant and obvious impairment of performance (see Appendix 2). Of note, from an experimental point of view, there has historically been great variability between laboratories and clinics in the protocols employed for the antisaccade task, which can of course greatly affect interpretation of results and make it difficult to compare conclusions from different studies. A useful 'harmonised' protocol for anti-saccades has therefore been suggested to help solve this issue, with some success to date (Antoniades, Ettinger et al. 2013).

Despite the complexity of the task, it turns out to be relatively easy to predict both the number of errors and the distribution of both antisaccade and prosaccade latencies by building on the kind of economical assemblies of small numbers of LATER units that are so successful in the case of tasks such as countermanding, Wheeless, or Go/ NoGo, where similar mistakes are frequently made. The key feature in all these cases is once again the Stop unit that cancels an ongoing decision process that has not yet reached its threshold (Figure 4.33(c)), whose existence is proved by the substantial gap between the distribution for error prosaccades and correct antisaccades (Figure 4.33(b), though this has been denied (Cutsuridis, Smyrnis et al. 2007). This gap between distributions is not explained simply by a time delay between two LATER units initiating, and hence implies the existence of another active (Stop) decision process. In the case of antisaccades, two other LATER units are responsible respectively for triggering the correct antisaccade (an Anti unit) and the incorrect prosaccade (a Pro unit). As can be seen in Figure 4.33(a), the appearance of the stimulus initiates both these units. The Anti unit is triggered after a delay representing the time needed to make the necessary spatial transformation from the actual location of the stimulus to the intended destination on the other side. The Stop unit is triggered at the same time: if it is fast enough, it cancels the Pro unit (Noorani and Carpenter 2013). Prior probability can be seen to have a large effect on the distributions. Another feature of

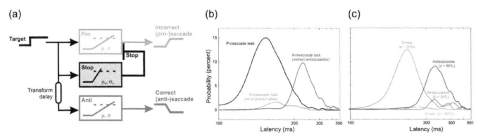

Figure 4.33 Modelling antisaccades. (a) A model for antisaccades, using two Go units for (correct) antisaccades and (erroneous) prosaccades. (b) Splined raw distributions from one subject (shown also as cumulative distributions in Figure 4.30(a)), emphasising the rightward shift of the antisaccade distribution relative to both the controls and error prosaccades. (c) Splined raw distributions for 80% prior probability and for 20%. Modified, after Noorani and Carpenter (2013).

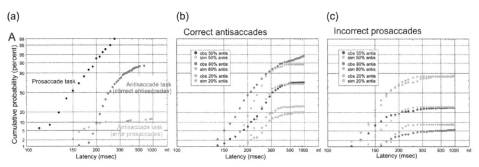

Figure 4.34 Distributions for the antisaccade task. (a) One subject's responses in a control (prosaccade) task (black), and for correct antisaccades and incorrect prosaccades. (b and c) Observed and simulated distributions for correct and incorrect responses, with different prior probabilities (20% and 80%), which can be seen to have a big effect, particularly on the final error rate. Note that these are incomplete distributions, showing cumulative probability as a fraction of all the trials. Modified from Noorani and Carpenter (2013).

this task is that subjects typically correct themselves after an error: that is, they look in the correct direction after initially looking the wrong way. The reaction times of these later correct responses can be easily modelled by employing a LATER Go unit that is only triggered on completion of an error by the first Go unit (Noorani and Carpenter 2014). In this way, the LATER model accurately recapitulates all major behaviours in the antisaccade task with remarkable simplicity, Figure 4.34.

LATER and the Brain

An act which may seem simple even to banality is the directing of the gaze. Yet its factors engage the roof-brain far and wide ...
Charles Sherrington, Man on his Nature *(1940)*

Structurally, the human brain is a mess. The problem is the way in which it has evolved: the bulk of what fills our skulls – the telencephalon, and especially the cerebral cortex – is relatively new, but it has not displaced the older and simpler structures seen in reptiles. Rather, the brain has evolved through *accretion* (Sarnat and Netsky 1974) (Figure 5.1): the older areas are still functional – indeed they are much the more important – but they have come to be supplemented and regulated by the newer areas, which provide improved overall integration and prediction through the massive bands of associational fibres that link every part of cerebral cortex to every other. In addition, these newer and 'higher' areas send and receive huge nerve tracts that have elbowed the older structures aside and distorted their shapes, making the relationships between their parts hard to discern. The key to understanding the structure of the brain is to think comparatively (Kaas 2009) – trying to identify in the human brain the fundamental components seen in simpler animals – and from a functional point of view to think hierarchically (Hughlings Jackson 1884), recognising the different roles played by the successive layers that have been laid down in the course of evolution.

In the case of saccades, this approach is particularly successful, as there is an obvious correlation between the anatomical levels (of which there are essentially three: hindbrain, midbrain, and cerebral cortex) and the intrinsic functional hierarchy that follows from the logic of what is needed to create eye movements to look at objects of importance

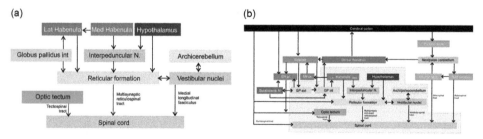

Figure 5.1 Evolution by accretion. (a) Schematic diagram of the motor system of a lower vertebrate. (b) Motor system of a typical mammal. The older system is essentially still present (grey area), but under the overall control of newer areas, particularly the cerebral cortex. Based on Sarnat and Netsky (1974).

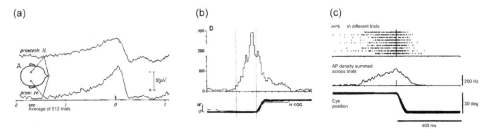

Figure 5.2 Slow build-up of activity long in advance of start of movement. (a) *Bereitschaftpotentialen* (Kornhuber and Deecke 1965); (b) parietal activity (Lynch, Mountcastle et al. 1977); (c) superior colliculus (Munoz and Wurtz 1995).

('how', 'where', and 'what' (Carpenter 2000, 2004)). In the introduction that follows, we start by outlining the evolutionary history, and then look at how this is reflected in the functional and anatomical hierarchy of the saccadic system. Undoubtedly, similar hierarchies exist for other motor systems, but they are not so clear. As Sherrington noted (Sherrington 1940), the saccadic system is almost a microcosm of the brain as a whole, but simpler because the final output is so much less complex.

Behavioural experiments are all very well, but never quite convincing to a neurophysiologist if they have no connection with observed neural activity. In fact, many groups of neurons in the brain show patterns of activity that resemble the main features of LATER. Over 50 years ago, Kornhuber and Deecke (1965) demonstrated by averaging evoked potentials in relation to spontaneous human actions that voluntary actions were preceded by a linear build-up of activity over several hundreds of milliseconds, the well-known (*Bereitschaftpotentialen* or readiness potentials, Figure 5.2). Subsequently, similar linear rises were demonstrated by intracellular recording in parietal cortex (Lynch, Mountcastle et al. 1977), in cerebellum (Llinas 1974, Noda, Asoh et al. 1977), and specifically saccade-related build-up activity was shown in superior colliculus (Schiller and Koerner 1971, Schiller and Stryker 1972, Wurtz and Goldberg 1972). Hanes and Schall (1996) showed that the activity of a class of movement-related neurons in the frontal eye fields (FEF) began to rise steadily before a saccade, that the initiation of the saccade was associated with this activity reaching a fixed threshold, and that the rate of rise varies randomly from trial to trial and was tightly correlated with the observed saccadic latency: all key features of LATER. Clearly, we need now to turn to the brain itself.

5.1 The Cerebral Hierarchy

Everything starts with the hollow, fluid-filled neural tube created by pinching off from the dorsal epithelium that forms the primitive nervous system. Sensory nerves from the skin enter it on the dorsal side, motor fibres leave on the ventral side; in between are fibres connecting it with the viscera. This threefold organisation – sensory, visceral, motor – from back to belly persists throughout evolution and can still be discerned even in the fully evolved human brain (Figure 5.3).

The second axis of polarisation is from head to tail (Figure 5.4). It clearly makes sense to develop specialised receptors in the head that will give advance warning of what is about to be encountered, and the processing of information from these receptors is generally more complex than what is required from the skin. Eyes generate spatial

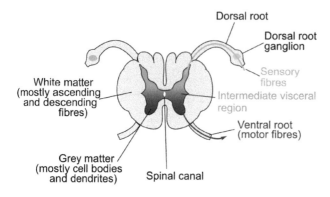

Figure 5.3 Schematic cross section of human neural tube, showing the regions associated with sensory, visceral, and motor nerve fibres. Modified from Carpenter and Reddi (2012).

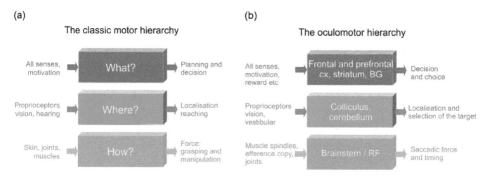

Figure 5.4 Functional and structural motor hierarchies. (a) For motor control in general; (b) specifically for the oculomotor system. cx, cortex; BG, basal ganglia; RF, reticular formation.

patterns of activity that need to be decoded, as do the temporal patterns from the ears; and all these senses need to be correlated with one another to make coherent sense of the outside world. As a result, the front end of the neural tube expands dramatically, with large clumps of neurons arranged in layers and in nuclei, carrying out these different kinds of computation. This expansion is partly the result of the dilation of the fluid-filled central canal to form large caverns, the ventricles. As we ascend from the spinal cord, we come to the fourth ventricle, followed by the third ventricle; this in turn generates a pair of lateral spurs, forming a Y, that then expand into the first and second, or lateral, ventricles (Figure 5.4). These three ventricular levels provide a classification of the neural structures that cluster round them: the region around the fourth ventricle is the hindbrain (pons and medulla), around the third ventricle is the midbrain (essentially, thalamus, tectum / colliculi) and the level of the lateral ventricles defines the forebrain (cerebral cortex, corpus striatum, hypothalamus, olfactory bulb).

In broad terms, these three levels have distinct, hierarchical functions (Hughlings Jackson 1884). At the lowest level, in the hindbrain, incoming information from the skin and from the vestibular system enables the animal to orient itself in space and generate the coordinated patterns of motor activity needed for locomotion. These functions must to a large extent be learnt, and this seems to have prompted the development of the cerebellum, an unusually regular computational structure that seems ideally suited to these kinds of learning. The primitive midbrain is dominated by the optic tectum (colliculus in higher animals) that appears to act as a centre for bringing different kinds of spatially patterned sensory information into relation with one another and for providing commands that descend to the lower motor areas to select appropriately directed movements. The forebrain, whose development seems to have been prompted by the massive inflow from the olfactory organs that is characteristic of more primitive animals, seems to be concerned not so much with spatial relationships but with recognition of stimuli, whether they are prey to be attacked and ingested or predators to be shunned. As Lord Balfour once put it (1914), '*The human brain is as much an organ for seeking food as the pig's snout.*' To do this, it needs to know about the body's homeostatic needs, through the all-important hypothalamus, with its afferent and efferent links with the homeostatic systems of the body, partly through nervous connections, partly through direct monitoring of the state of the blood, and partly through the hormones that it controls through the pituitary, and with links to primitive cortical regions – archicortex – that enable it to learn from experience whether, for instance, a particular morsel was good to eat or not.

We then end up with a hierarchy that is at the same time both anatomical and functional, which can be summarised as *What*, *Where*, and *How* (Figure 5.4).

Figure 5.5 represents these functional relationships in a very simplified form, side by side with an outline of the anatomy of one particular primitive brain that happens to have been studied in particular detail, the tiger salamander, *Ambystoma tigrinum* (Kaas 2009). Though this basic ground-plan can be discerned in the human brain, the biggest single difference is that our forebrain is massively expanded by the development of neocortex (it has six layers rather than the three of archicortex). In the course of evolution, its surface area grows dramatically, throwing it into the well-known folds and furrows that enable a large area of cortex to be packed into a relatively small skull. As a result, practically nothing can be seen of the human brain except the cortex and cerebellum and part of the brainstem (Figure 5.5).

5.1.1 Superior Colliculus

The superior colliculus is a downstream motor output of key eye movement brain regions including the FEF. There are groups of neurons in the superior colliculus that are more active during visual fixation (fixation neurons) or during saccades (saccade neurons), and there are lateral inhibitory connections between these neurons in the intermediate layers of the ipsilateral and contralateral superior colliculus. These connections help to prevent saccades to unwanted targets and to maintain stable visual fixation.

The superior colliculus was once thought to represent a simple motor region that follows commands from the higher cerebral regions where decisions on eye movements are made. However, more recent work has challenged this assumption, and has posited the superior colliculus to be actively involved in decision-making for where to look or at least to be part of a distributed neural network that makes such decisions (Krauzlis and Dill 2002). There is some neurophysiological evidence to support this concept, provided by neural recording studies in monkeys. For example, reducing the probability of a visual target appearing led to reduced baseline activity of groups of neurons in the superior colliculus of monkeys; these neurons were responsive to visual targets appearing without any delays; when the probability of target appearance was reduced, the activity of these neurons further predicted saccadic latency (Basso and Wurtz 1998). These results are consistent with such neurons representing a LATER decision-making unit, with the reduction in baseline neural activity coincident with reduced target probability reflecting a reduced S_0 of the LATER unit.

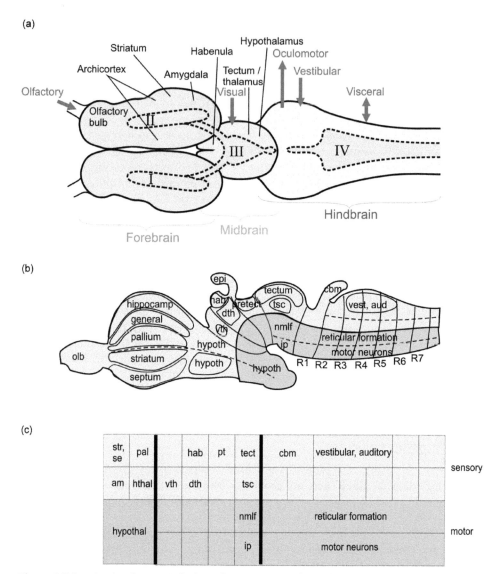

Figure 5.5 Functional and anatomical relationships in a primitive brain (the tiger salamander). (a) Schematic dorsal view, showing the three main divisions. (b) The internal organisation. (c) Highly schematised representation. Data from Kaas (2009). am, amygdala; cbm, cerebellum; dlt, dorsolateral tegmentum; dth, vth, dorsal and ventral thalamus; hab, habenula; ip, interpeduncular nuclei; lc, locus coeruleus; na, nucleus accumbens; nmlf, nucleus of the medial longitudinal fasciculus; nr, raphe nucleus; pal, pallium; pt, pretectum; se, septum; sn, substantia nigra; str, striatum; tsc, torus semicircularis; vt ventral tegmentum.

5.1.2 Basal Ganglia

The basal ganglia receive many inputs from cortical regions and send outputs to cortex and brainstem, necessary for the role of the basal ganglia in planning and generating movements. With regards to eye movements, the basal ganglia have connections with higher regions including the FEF and with the superior colliculus. Its inhibitory connections with the superior colliculus are tonically active, such that they prevent initiation of saccades to unwanted targets. More recent experiments have supported the importance of the basal ganglia in stopping movements. Stopping, where one must cancel an impending movement, is an often-underestimated aspect of movement control. Imagine sitting in your car: as the traffic lights turn green, you are about to step on the accelerator when a pedestrian starts walking in front of you – you must stop what you are about to do to avoid hurting them! This plan to stop a movement represents a special type of decision for the brain, and as such we proposed that stopping is generated by a special Stop decision LATER unit. Just like any other LATER unit, it races towards a threshold; unlike other LATER units, however, if it wins a race with other LATER units, the Stop unit will pause a movement rather than generating one. The Stop unit was shown to be crucial for explaining decision times in the anti-saccade, Wheeless, and Go / NoGo tasks, as elaborated on previously.

It is widely believed that basal ganglia function as two opposing pathways, namely, the direct and indirect pathways. This idea has helped us understand clinical motor deficits seen in neurological disorders related to basal ganglia pathology, such as Parkinson's disease and Huntington's disease. The direct pathway has an inhibitory output; the pathway goes from the striatum to the globus pallidus internus and substantia nigra (SNpr); increased activity in this pathway leads to reduced output. The indirect pathway has an excitatory output and runs from the striatum to the globus pallidus externus, thence to the subthalamic nucleus (STN), and from there to the globus pallidus internus and substantia nigra. Movement can therefore be triggered or suppressed by altering the balance between these two pathways of the basal ganglia. It is conceivable that the basal ganglia can also control the stopping of movement by means of a race to threshold between competing pathways. Indeed, neurophysiological recordings in brains of rodents that were performing a Go / NoGo task has suggested exactly this. In this experiment, in trials presenting the Stop signal to the rodent, the STN became active just after presentation of that signal, regardless of whether the subsequent movement was successfully cancelled or not. On the other hand, downstream neurons of the SNpr were active only in trials with successful movement cancellation. This implies the existence of a pathway from STN to SNpr that can cancel impending movements. On trials where the rodent was instructed to move without a Stop signal, there was increased input from striatum to SNpr, suggesting this pathway drives Go movements (Schmidt, Leventhal et al. 2013). Thus, the ability of the rodent to cancel a movement depends on a race between these two pathways, with the winning pathway providing the dominant input to the SNpr on that trial (and thus determining whether the movement is cancelled). One could argue this experimental demonstration represents the LATER model in action in the brain! It is not too difficult to imagine such races between Go and Stop in the basal ganglia explaining behaviour in other Stop tasks such as anti-saccades (Noorani and Carpenter 2014).

5.1.3 Habenula

The habenula forms part of the epithalamus, which also includes the pineal body: it consists of two distinct nuclei – lateral and medial (Sarnat and Netsky 1974, Bianco and Wilson 2009, Aizawa, Amo et al. 2011). The medial nucleus projects to the lateral and is the origin of the main output from the habenula to the interpeduncular nucleus.

Corresponding to its commanding position right at the top of the primitive brain, it seems to have many of the same global decision-making functions as the areas that have superseded it (Figure 5.1). In particular, it is the source of tonic dopaminergic descending inhibition, temporarily and locally lifted to permit a specified response to take place. As a result, when lesioned, exploratory and other spontaneous behaviour tends to increase (Bianco and Wilson 2009). Its activity is hugely determined by reward, being inhibited by stimuli that predict reward and stimulated by those associated with lack of reward. These features are reminiscent of the behaviour of dopaminergic neurons in substantia nigra pars compacta, except that the latter are the other way round, increasing their activity when rewards are greater than expected, and reducing it when they are less (Schultz 2000, 2007, 2016). The habenula also contributes to the evaluation of and response to pain , with an important projection from the lateral nucleus to brainstem structures such as the raphe nucleus and peri-aqueductal grey that modify the perception of painful stimuli (Shelton, Beccerra et al. 2012).

5.1.4 Frontal Eye Fields

The frontal eye fields (FEF) are at the top of the hierarchy for saccadic movements and decisions. There is an important descending projection to the superior colliculus, providing information about visual stimuli; but most have no saccade-related activity (Ferraina, Paré et al. 2002). There are also neurons in the FEF whose activity correlates with that of an eye movement; these are rather unsurprisingly called 'movement neurons'. The FEF is discussed in general reviews elsewhere (Schall, Hanes et al. 1995, Schall, Stuphorn et al. 2002, Schall 2004). A key concept of the LATER model that explains the variability in reaction times is that of randomness in the rate of rise of LATER activity towards the threshold. An important test to validate the accuracy of this model therefore is to determine whether neurons controlling decisions actually display such randomly variable behaviour. This can be done by neuronal recordings in FEF (specifically the movement neurons) of monkeys whilst the animals are making saccadic eye movement. So, what does this experiment tell us? After a visual stimulus is presented, neural activity in these FEF movement neurons begins to rise following a short delay, and when the saccade movement starts, the activity of these neurons collapses (Hanes and Schall 1996). Also (and very satisfyingly!), the activity of these neurons rises at a different rate from trial to trial, and this variability is indeed random around a constant mean value, consistent with the LATER model concept. Moreover, the starting neural activity and threshold for saccade initiation do not vary in this random manner for the movement neurons. So, at first glance it would appear that there are indeed neural correlates of the LATER model units in the brain that behave in the way the model predicts.

We mentioned before that their response time distributions and their modelling suggests the existence of two separate neural stages in responses: a stimulus detection stage followed by a decision stage. But what is the evidence that the brain actually responds with two such discrete stages? Further recordings in the FEF reveal another group of neurons that are active in a way more related to the onset of a visual stimulus than a subsequent eye movement. When recording these 'sensory' neurons in monkeys performing an 'oddball' task (where they must discriminate between balls based on their colour), we find that the sensory neurons increase their activity on presentation of a stimulus regardless of whether that stimulus has the correct colour or not. After a certain delay, corresponding to the time needed for processing of colour information in the cerebral cortex, the sensory neuronal activity drops if the ball colour is wrong, but continues to rise sharply if it is the right colour. At this moment when the sensory neuronal activity is high after colour information arrives, the movement neurons begin to increase their activity. Interestingly, the time taken for the sensory neuron activity to rise towards a threshold or collapse if the target is the wrong colour is relatively constant and therefore not correlated with the random variability of the final reaction times. All of these experiments point to the same clear conclusion: the origin of the randomness in reaction times must not lie in the first detection stage or any noisiness of the incoming sensory stimuli, but rather it is due to the brain having inherent variability in the second stage where the rate of rise of movement neuronal activity varies from trial to trial. The brain is creating its own randomness!

5.1.5 Supplementary Eye Field

In addition to the FEF, the supplementary eye field (SEF) is another region of the frontal lobe that is critical for eye movements and decisions to make them (Nachev, Kennard et al. 2008). The FEF and SEF are strongly interconnected and share a lot of their input, and project to similar areas (Carpenter 2004), Figure 5.6. Certain movements require subjects to learn a new association between a stimulus and their response, for example, in the antisaccade task the subject must learn to look in the opposite direction to that of the

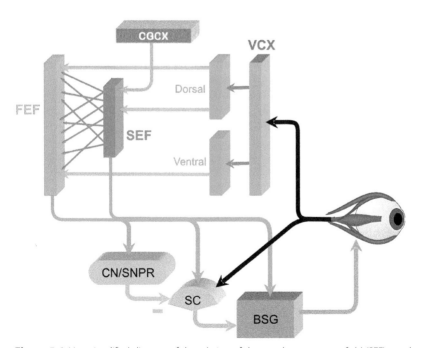

Figure 5.6 Very simplified diagram of the relation of the supplementary eye field (SEF) to other oculomotor areas: note than many of the connections are partly reciprocal. CGCX, cingulate cortex; CN/SNPR, caudate nucleus and substantia nigra pars reticulata; FEF, frontal eye fields; VCX, visual cortical areas, with dorsal ('where') and ventral ('what') streams; BSG, brainstem circuits generating saccades; SC superior colliculus.

stimulus. Studies have shown that SEF neurons can alter their firing when such associations are being learnt, and are also more active prior to making anti-saccades than pro-saccades, thus implicating the SEF in complex voluntary decision processes. The SEF may also have an even higher role in behaviour, as supported by its mutual connections with the cingulate cortex – it may act as a kind of 'moral system', at least for eye movements, whereby it monitors performance and behaviour, responding to mistakes accordingly. People performing the countermanding task, for example, often have temporary feelings of guilt after making an error, reflected in a short-lived increase in reaction times where the subject becomes more cautious in subsequent responses. In this way, it is thought the SEF oversees our behaviour at a high level and sets the tone for giving our best performance, at least in such tasks as countermanding and antisaccades.

5.1.6 Lateral Intraparietal Area

A major assumption of the LATER model for decision-making is that neurons that control the decision process represent the log likelihood ratio of a potential choice or response. This has been investigated using animal models, providing some useful insight. For example, in one study monkeys were trained to perform a probabilistic reward task, in which the monkeys had to choose between a pair of coloured targets after watching a sequence of four shapes that signal which of the upcoming targets is most likely to provide the monkeys with a reward. By recording from neurons in the lateral intraparietal area (LIP), the investigators were able to show that these neurons respond in a way that is akin to an accumulation towards a threshold for a behavioural choice; moreover, firing rates of these neurons correlated with the log likelihood ratio (LLR) (as derived from the sequence of shapes presented to the monkeys) (Yang and Shadlen 2007). Regarding potential neural correlates of the LATER correlates, a controversial area is precisely how neurons may be accumulating evidence towards a threshold. Recordings from single neurons in the LIP of monkeys revealed that these neurons displayed a 'spiking' behaviour, wherein their firing rate jumped from one value to another, reflecting an essentially digital rather than analogue form of neural implementation of decision behaviour (Latimer, Yates et al. 2015). As we have alluded to, a decision, however, would be generated through activity from a pool of neurons rather than any one neuron in particular, rather like a committee coming to a joint decision instead of a leader making a unilateral decision.

5.1.7 Cingulate Cortex

Given that decision-making in the brain is likely generated through large neural networks rather than solely individual areas, it is worth mentioning the role of other cortical areas. We previously discussed how altering the predictive information about a stimulus to a subject affects their reaction times: in particular, there is a swivel in the reaction time distributions, which would be accounted for by a change in the distance to threshold of the decision process rather than a change in the rate of rise. A study with human subjects performing a Go / NoGo task altered the predictive information provided about upcoming stimuli, confirming a swivel in the reaction time distributions. This study went further by using functional magnetic resonance imaging (fMRI) to show that the anterior cingulate cortex was the only area of the brain whose activity correlated with the subject's ability to use predictive information to appropriately modulate the distance to threshold of the decision process (Dolmenech and Dreher 2010). Moreover, fMRI techniques suggested that this region feeds information in the dorsolateral prefrontal cortex where neural correlates of the decision signal itself were apparent. This study highlights how the decision process is reliant on several distributed brain regions all working together as part of a neural network.

5.2 The Need for Ascending Control

We have known for over 50 years that the cortex is under relatively diffuse control by ascending innervation having its origin mostly in the brainstem, a discovery that seemed to make good functional sense. Clearly, there is a need for the general level of activity of the brain to be regulated both in different generalised states of arousal and in correspondence with local attention.

When, more recently, it became clear that this was not a single system but consists of four or possibly five separate divisions, associated with different neurotransmitters (noradrenaline, NA; serotonin, 5HT; dopamine, DA; acetylcholine, ACh; and perhaps histamine) and originating from a variety of nuclei in the brainstem and elsewhere, it became apparent that the simple view that these systems were simply for 'arousal' would not do (Robbins 1997, Robbins, Granon et al. 1998, Robbins 2000), Figure 5.7.

A set of four or five distinct regulatory functions was needed that might correspond with these chemically and anatomically distinct systems. There has been much effort to try to identify what these functions might be (Everitt and Robbins 1997, Robbins 1997, Robbins, Granon et al. 1998, Robbins 2000), and some interesting conclusions have emerged, necessarily of a somewhat tentative and general kind. The NA system seems most likely to be associated with 'attention' in the classic sense, possibly acting to raise the activity of selected inputs while suppressing competing ones. The 5HT pathways may perhaps be regarded as acting more on the output of the cortical system, altering reactivity and causing the well-known effects on spontaneous movement.

The DA system seems to be associated with motivation and response evaluation. ACh appears specifically to regulate the relative weighting attached to new and old information, in effect the relative contribution of stored models and actual incoming information (Yu and Dayan 2005, Goard and Dan 2009, Smythies 2009) (see Section 3.7). About histamine we have the least information, and it remains something of a mystery.

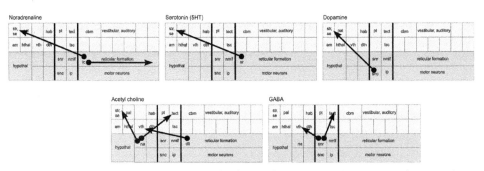

Figure 5.7 Various ascending systems associated with particular transmitters. (Gamma-aminobutyric acid (GABA) is not 'ascending' in this sense, but is included for completeness). Highly simplified and schematic, as in Figure 5.5, where a list of the abbreviations can be found. Data from Nieuwenhuys (1985).

A bold and quite attractive conjecture about why we have several different ascending systems is that in a decision-making system like LATER there are several parameters that may have to be differently adjusted in different circumstances. It would be natural, for instance, to associate the NA system with control of the starting level of the decision signal: attention is after all not very different from expectation or prior probability. To the extent that it might alter the degree of variability (σ) in LATER (Aron, Schlagheeken et al. 2002, Aron, Fletcher et al. 2003, Aron, Sahakian et al. 2003), it could fulfil the essential role of keeping creativity under control: when foraging, trying new strategies is to be welcomed – when crossing Niagara Falls on a tightrope, less so. The general characteristics of the 5HT system suggest that it might control the output threshold for action; and the cholinergic system might conceivably alter the balance between information stored as neural models, and the actual incoming information, influencing the relative weighting given by LATER, to new information versus stored experience, Figure 5.8.

Motivation and evaluation of response, where DA would be expected to have most influence, is not yet part of the formal LATER model (but see Section 6.3), though it is currently an active area of study. It is not clear whether the system decides what is 'true' and then, as a separate operation, decides a response on the basis of utility, or whether the value of a response actually feeds into the LATER model itself. Lauwereyns et al. (2002) suggest the latter, and that perceived value scales the decision signal, Figure 5.9.

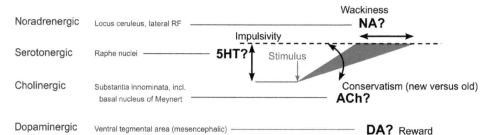

Figure 5.8 Highly schematic representation of how the four main ascending systems might be used specifically to regulate different aspects of LATER's behaviour. NA, noradrenaline; 5HT, serotonin; Ach, acetylcholine; DA, dopamine.

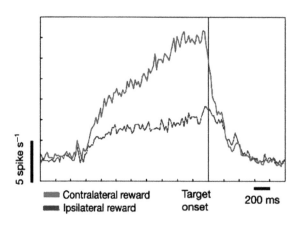

Figure 5.9 Electrical responses from monkey caudate nucleus in a task in which the monkey made a saccade in every trial, but was rewarded for a correct response in only half of the trials, depending on the position of the visual target (Lauwereyns, Watanabe et al. 2002). Neurons usually fire more (red) when contralateral reward is expected, with decreased latency for eye movements in the contralateral direction.

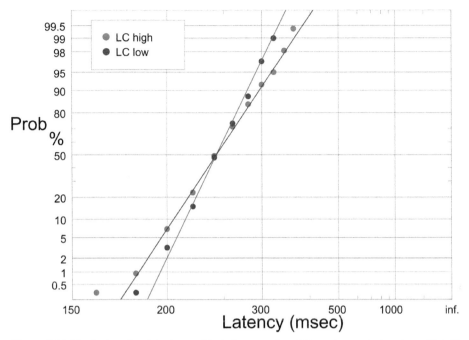

Figure 5.10 Distributions for trials when activity in locus ceruleus (LC) was low, and when it was high. The activity appears to correlate with a pure change in the LATER parameter σ. (Usher, Cohen et al. 1999).

Over recent years, a number of papers have been published, using widely diverging techniques and coming from groups with very different backgrounds and assumptions, that provide some grounds for thinking that this approach might be fruitful. They include studies that link reaction time and decision tasks to different ascending systems and the neuroactive substances associated with them – most specifically, Aron's work (Aron, Schlagheeken et al. 2002, Aron, Fletcher et al. 2003, Aron, Sahakian et al. 2003) on countermanding; others that link alterations in reaction time (RT) distributions to attention-deficit/hyperactivity disorder (ADHD) (Leth-Steensen, Elbaz et al. 2000, Munoz, Armstrong et al. 2003), and fluctuations in RT to different forms of dementia, and, particularly interestingly, Usher's finding (Usher, Cohen et al. 1999) that alterations in activity of the locus ceruleus appear to be associated with changes in just a single LATER parameter (σ), Figure 5.10.

5.3 The Source of Randomness

Recording from stimulus-related cells in frontal eye fields in tasks requiring one stimulus to be discriminated from another do indeed show randomness in the time taken to make the discrimination. But when contrasts are high, its contribution to the overall variability of reaction time is insignificant (Schall and Bichot 1998). (See Section 4.6.2). This implies that the observed randomness of reaction time does not originate in the outside world, or even in the intrinsic noise in our sensory receptors. Rather, it is gratuitously – deliberately – injected into the system from within.

At first sight, this seems a crazy thing for the brain to do. What possible advantage could there be in making the timing of our responses more random than they need be?

Of course, one might well think that whether a response sometimes takes 150 ms and sometimes 250 ms simply doesn't matter very much. But there is one reason why in fact it matters a great deal. If we race between a number of competing hypotheses, any randomness of response time gets translated into something much more important, randomness of *which* response is finally chosen. The consequence is profound: even if all the factors surrounding a particular trial are held constant, on different occasions different LATER units may happen to win. *Randomness of timing results in randomness of choice.*

5.3.1 Implementing Randomness

We have seen that randomness seems to be injected gratuitously into the decision-making system; but how is it generated? There are three distinct possibilities: it could be generated independently in individual neurons, or it could be the result of some kind of overall randomiser, perhaps projecting up from the brainstem, or it could be the consequence of chaotic behaviour characteristic of complex networks of interacting elements, Figure 5.11.

5.3.2 Cellular

When we present a subject with a pair of targets, on the left and on the right, separated in time by d ms (a *precedence* task: see Section 4.5.1), we find that although there is a tendency, increasing with increasing d to make a saccade to the first of the pair that appeared (Leach and Carpenter 2001), the choice is stochastic: very often the saccade will be made to the second target rather than the first. The implication is profound: the variability in the rate of rise of the decision must be *independent* in the two LATER units. If it were not, and common to both units, then whichever target appears first will inevitably be the final destination, and the other will never be chosen.

That individual bacteria are capable of making random movements is clear when comparing their two-dimensional tracks with those made by saccades when scanning static scenes (Brockman and Geisel 1999, Brockman and Geisel 2000, Reynolds 2007). Furthermore, it is clear that at least some bacteria have complex enough internal

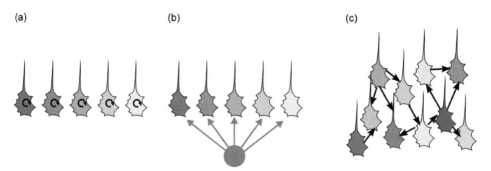

(a)   (b)   (c)

Figure 5.11 Generic ways of creating randomness. (a) *Intracellular:* each neuron has an independent, built-in randomiser that is independent of the others. (b) *Extracellular* randomness: an ascending projection (blue) randomly modulates each of a set of neurons. (c) *Emergent* randomness: the randomness in the activity is due to an emergent property of the chaos characteristic of neural networks.

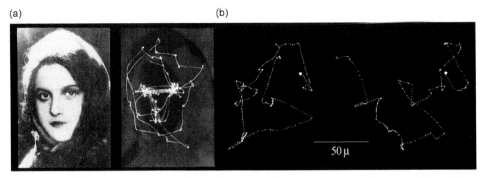

Figure 5.12 (a) Saccadic trajectories while scanning a face; (b) tracks made by motile bacteria (Yarbus 1967, Berg and Brown 1972).

machinery to be capable of implementing simple decisions, including those with stochastic elements (Bray 2009), Figure 5.12.

5.3.3 Externally Generated Randomness

The notion of ascending projections from the brainstem whose activity is stochastic and in effect drive the random component of LATER units is an obvious one. But it is ruled out by the precedence experiments just described, and would also be purposeless, since the whole point is to have units whose randomness is independent of each other. In any case, no such projections have ever been described, though – as we have seen – there is some evidence for ascending systems that regulate the degree of randomness, which is not at all the same thing as actually generating it (Usher, Cohen et al. 1999).

5.3.4 Emergent Chaotic Behaviour

A chaotic system is one that generates superficially random behaviour that turns out on closer examination to be quasi-periodic; in other words, when restarted with the original parameters it behaves exactly as it did the first time. To the extent that its behaviour may nevertheless be essentially unpredictable, under the right conditions it can look like a randomiser, especially as such systems are in general particularly sensitive to very small changes in the initial conditions.

While it is fairly clear that the neural networks within the brain have all the properties – massive self-interactions, and especially distributive feedback loops – that would make them likely candidates for generating chaotic behaviour, despite much early enthusiasm it has to be said that the amount of well-supported evidence that chaotic behaviour plays a role in randomising decision-making has been disappointing (May 1976, Yoshimatsu and Yamada 1991, Abadi, Broomhead et al. 1997, Stam 2005).

5.4 Attention

'Attention' is one of those vague words that is best avoided. Is it a causative agent rather than a retrospective description of behaviour? Many neurons in decision-linked systems do show alterations in their background rate of firing that are often associated with situations where a human would report that they were attending to a stimulus. But they show similar fluctuations in response to prior probability, and since there can only be

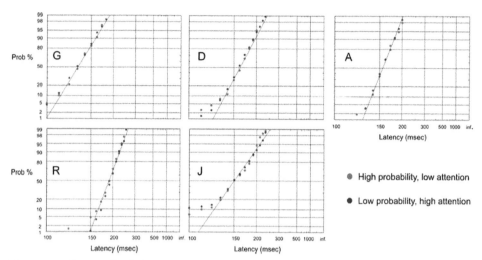

Figure 5.13 Titration of probability against attention. Latency distributions for five subjects, for targets that were either more attended but less expected, or more expected but less attended. In each case, the distributions are statistically indistinguishable (Kolmogorov-Smirnov, $pG = 0.14$, $pD = 0.14$, $pA = 0.56$, $pR = 0.50$, $pJ = 0.73$). Note the small number of early saccades for some subjects, with equal incidence in the two cases. Roger Carpenter, unpublished data.

one rate of background firing, it seems likely that at some level prior probability and attention are simply the same thing. Since probability can actually be quantified, whereas attention cannot, it is more useful to describe the phenomenon as a kind of expectation rather than attention.

One way of demonstrating this is to interleave trials using attention to heighten expectation that the target is in a particular location, with trials in which the same function is carried out by using a predictive cue to manipulate prior probability. In one such experiment, attention trials began with a central fixation target, which after a random foreperiod was supplemented with a pair of cues, red arrows pointing either left or right, with equal probability. After 500 ms, the cues were extinguished and the target jumped to the left or right. In prior probability trials, after the foreperiod all four arrows appeared for 500 ms, when they disappeared and the target jumped to left or right; the probability p of jumping left was constant throughout a run. We can then 'titrate' the two factors by varying their strengths until they produce identical distributions (Figure 5.13).

Larger Implications

The set of new techniques triggered an enormous explosion of research which has led – as explosions usually do – to the generation of numberless fragments ('data'), but not in itself any great gain in our understanding and insights.
Rudolph Nieuwenhuys, Chemoarchitecture of the Brain *(1985)*

6.1 What Is a Stimulus?

Of all the biological sciences, it is the study of the brain that most impinges on philosophy; and like philosophers, neuroscientists need to take special care in how they name things (Smythies 2009). Most would agree that the function of the brain is to convert stimuli into responses. But what is a stimulus? Is it best considered as the pattern formed by the combined activity of all sensory receptors at a given point in time? That is indeed what ultimately determines what the brain does. But it is not at all what is being described, for instance, in the Methods section of scientific papers. Here 'stimulus' means something extremely localised and specific – perhaps a dot of a certain size and colour – and there is tacit complicity with the subject that nothing else counts in making the response that is to be measured. There is also complicity regarding which aspects of the stimulus will be quietly ignored. Some will be quite different on different occasions, depending on the lighting conditions and where the subject happens to be looking. The sensory pattern is the product of the *intrinsic* properties of the 'stimulus' and *accidental* features that continually vary. Indeed, an important function – some would say the only function – of sensory systems is generalisation: working out which sensory patterns are in fact to be treated as 'the same' because they are due to a particular 'stimulus' (Pirenne 1950). This much is a commonplace of current received opinion, yet we still persist in using 'stimulus' to mean these two quite different things: the sensory pattern (that we might perhaps call afference), and the thing in the outside world to which we are invited to respond, which we might call the object. In perception, what we are trying to perceive is the original object that generates the stimuli that impinge on our senses, and these stimuli must in turn have accidental aspects stripped from them in order to reveal what is intrinsic to the object. A good example is the perception of colour. When we look at a reflective object, the spectrum of the light entering our eyes is partly a function of the spectrum of the reflectance of the object (essential), and partly of the spectrum of the illumination (accidental). Much of the adaptational functions of the visual system are devoted to deciding which is which (Carpenter and Reddi 2012).

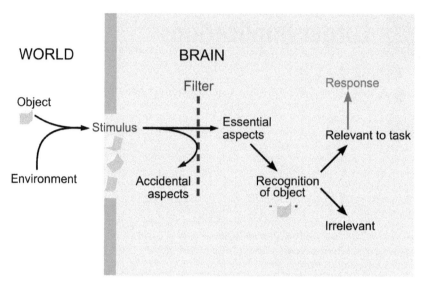

Figure 6.1 An object in the environment generates a retinal image (a stimulus), but some of its attributes are accidental (viewing angle, for example) rather than essential. The first stage of visual processing is recognition of the object by means of these essential attributes. But not all of the essential attributes of the object are needed to perform the task; the Irrelevant ones are (temporarily) ignored.

This is of course the notion of the Platonic ideal – the whatness of all-horse (Joyce 1922). But we would argue that it is necessary to go one stage further again in this process of generalisation, that what must be identified is not the object, but the action that the object implies: what Merleau-Ponty (1945) calls 'affordances'. If several objects require the same action, they can be grouped together as a single entity. What should the brain do to distinguish between them?

It is through the instructions given to a subject at the start of a run that they know what responses to make to certain stimuli. If they are told to saccade to a target dot, regardless of its colour, its detection leads directly to the appropriate action. That we do in fact perceive the colour of the dot, even when it was irrelevant to action, suggests that the brain does distinguish between stimuli, but that it does not delay action to resolve this distinction (Figure 6.1). This is probably because the information is used to evaluate outcomes. For instance, introducing a reward for one colour (when both are to be responded to) would be expected to lead to a change in reaction times and the stimuli being treated differently, despite the fact that the action required is the same. Perceptions could be defined in terms of what they can cause – if they have no consequences, they are not worth perceiving (Merleau-Ponty 1945). The same rule of survival of the best predictors works here too. Those that predict actions survive, as do those that predict stimuli.

6.2 Multidimensional Inference

The real world normally offers much more than just two possible targets. So, we need to think about *n*-dimensional probability-space. Can LATER cope? In principle, we can imagine a single point representing the current state of belief in each hypothesis, and that when information is received, the point moves to some new position. Information is

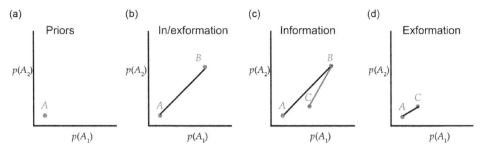

Figure 6.2 The difference between information and exformation. Starting with the prior probabilities (a), $p(A_1)$ and $p(A_2)$, we then receive a message purporting to update these values, B (b). But then a second message arrives, telling us the first message was wrong, and the true values are at C (c,d). From an internal point of view, we see a relatively long path-length (b); but externally the path-length is short, directly from A to C (c).

reduction in uncertainty: it must be closely related to movements in probability-space. But receiving information does not always reduce uncertainty: it does not have a sign. A probability changing from 0.5 to 0.9 is the same amount of information as changing from 0.5 to 0.1: furthermore, it is the same as changing from 0.9 to 0.5! Specifically, one message may nullify a previous message, perhaps directly telling us that it was false (Figure 6.2). Therefore, information must be related to something like path-length in probability space rather than being a vector. A message is indeed a vector, but its information content is not. Yet an observation that contradicts a previous one *does* in fact increase knowledge: one's confidence is increased, even if the probability has not changed. Paradoxically, if trajectory length is what matters, noisy channels convey more information than good ones, as the signals are more likely to contradict themselves.

In the simplest case, E is also multidimensional and consists entirely of sense-data S derived from the existence in the outside world of a set X of one or more of the n possible objects. That implies either that it is trained by knowing X independently of S, or alternatively that the brain forms its own categorisation of objects through mutual associations. There then have to be two processes (though they may turn out to be the same): a process Y that recognises stimulus clusters that are coherent objects, and a process Z that creates Y from comparison of S and E:Y is not given; it must be learnt. Clusters occur because they are caused by the same object – the basic problem is once more of separating the intrinsic and accidental features of a stimulus (Section 6.1) – those that occur together reinforce one other.

6.2.1 Complex Likelihood Ratios

Likelihood ratios need not be limited to comparisons of just two hypotheses. In two dimensions, likelihood ratio is equivalent to the direction of a vector; in n-dimensional space, it is still the direction of a vector; the same is true of odds. In three dimensions, complex odds/likelihood are analogous to the colour triangle: saturation is equivalent to strength of belief/evidence; hue to the most favoured hypothesis (or combination of hypotheses). The angle made with the unit vector would be a good measure of strength of belief: in fact it is related to Student's t-distribution (Sommerville 1958, Kendall 1961, Stoyan, Kendall et al. 1995, Wickens 1995, Saville and Wood 1996). If the probabilities/likelihoods are $x_1, x_2, \ldots, x_n$, then if μ is the mean and σ its SD, the required angle is simply $\arctan(\sigma/\mu)$. Neuronally, a more useful measure would be the set of angles made

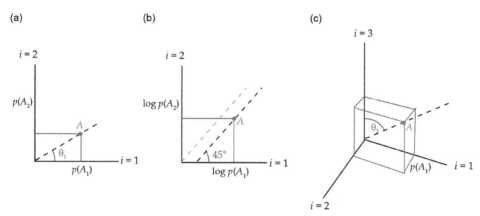

Figure 6.3 Graphical representation of complex probabilities. (a) linear axes, $N = 2$; (b) log axes, $N = 2$; (c) linear axes, $N = 3$.

with the various axes. This angle, for hypothesis k, is given by $\arccos(x_k/\sqrt{\Sigma(x_i^2)})$. Log likelihood ratio generalises even more easily to n dimensions – see above ($\mathscr{E} \log x - \log x_i$). Yet another geometrically attractive possibility is Distance in log-probability, $\sqrt{(\Sigma (\log(p_i'/p_i))^2)}$.

Very often in trying to make inferential judgements, one wants to know the *relative* probability of two possibilities to decide between them, but their *absolute* probabilities may not matter very much. When considering composite possibilities, it can be helpful to use the log-odds function, also known as rather ugly lod(X), or perhaps cred(X).

It is convenient at this point to introduce a geometrical representation of odds and their logs. Suppose we represent $p(A_1)$ and $p(A_2)$ in two dimensions by using a pair of orthogonal axes (Figure 6.3(a)). Then the odds are simply given by the slope of a line from the origin to a point $(p(A_1)/p(A_2))$ representing the two probabilities, and any point on that line correspond to pairs of probabilities having the same odds. This line makes an angle θ_1 with the $i = 1$ axis, where $\tan \theta_1 = p(A_2)/p(A_1)$. Alternatively, $\cos \theta_1 = p(A_1)/\sqrt{(p^2(A_1)^2 + p^2(A_2)^2)}$, which has the advantage that it lends itself to generalisation.

If linear, each axis could literally represent the probability of a hypothesis. If the axes exhaust the hypotheses, then there is a redundancy in that the current state X is necessarily constrained to a plane, since the sum of the components A_i is necessarily 1. On the other hand, many hypotheses will certainly not be mutually exclusive.

Alternatively, the components could be the number of favourable instances for each hypothesis. The direction of A will then represent the complex odds, and the amplitude $|A|$ will reflect the strength of the belief.

Alternatively, we can think in terms of log odds: now the line representing all pairs of probabilities having the same odds is represented by a line through $(\log p(A_1), \log p(A_2))$ and not through the origin, with a slope of 1. Its intercept with the $i = 1$ axis will represent the value of lod(A_1, A_2), and its distance from a parallel line projecting from the origin will be lod(A_1, A_2)^2. (Figure 6.3(b)).

So, we can see how to use odds or log odds to represent the relative probabilities of just two hypotheses, but in real life there may be *many* to be compared and from which to select the most likely. Can we extend the idea of odds to cases where the number of propositions, N, is more than two? The geometrical interpretation suggests an answer. Imagine first of all that $N = 3$, with a third proposition, A_3 (Figure 6.3(c)). We now have a three-dimensional space in which A is at the point $(pA_1, pA_2, pA_3,)$. Once again, a line from the origin through this point represents all the cases for which the odds between any pair of these probabilities are constant. Using the same notation as before, that the angle between this line and a given axis i is θ_i , we have $\cos \theta_i = p(A)/(p(A_i)/\sqrt{\Sigma p^2(A_i)}$. This essentially gives a measure of the degree to which one hypothesis, A_i, is to be preferred against all the alternatives: θ_i ranges from $0°$ to $90°$, with a small value denoting higher odds, and $45°$ means complete indifference, and these values apply whatever the number of alternatives.

We can derive a geometrical version of N-dimensional log odds in a similar way, using logarithmic axes for $\log p(A_1)$, $\log p(A_2)$, and so on. As before, a line with unit direction through A will represent all those combinations of probabilities having the same set of log odds. A useful measure of the degree to which a hypothesis A_i is preferred to the others is described by Kullback–Leibler (KL) divergence. The KL divergence is a measure of how different two probability distributions are from each other, and it can be used to quantify the degree to which one hypothesis is preferred over another. The KL divergence between be two hypotheses can be described as:

$$D_{\mathrm{KL}}(p(A_{i-}) \| p(A_i)) = \mathrm{E}[\log(p(A_{i-})/p(A_i))],$$

where D_{KL} denotes the KL divergence, $p(A_{i-})$ and $p(A_i)$ are probability distributions corresponding to two hypotheses (A_{i-} and A_i), and E denotes the expectation over some data distribution.

We shall see later that this measure of the credibility of a particular hypothesis lends itself particularly easily to implementation by networks of neurons.

Another kind of log representation is that the entire diagram could represent the contribution of events to belief in just one hypothesis. Each axis is then log likelihood (i.e., synaptic strength), and learning means a change in the position of A. For the amplitude A to mean something useful, each axis needs to be normalised as $\log(p(E|H)/p(E))$. In fact, the synapses themselves need to be normalised like this. If several different neurons are encoding different hypotheses on the same set of events, then each would be a separate point in this space – quite a useful representation. Then lateral inhibition between them should mutually repel the points – not just in direction but perhaps in length. The failures then get wiped clean – become more innocent – so they can be re-used.

6.2.2 Probability Vectors

The idea of N-dimensional odds as a vector has a number of virtues. It embodies the idea that combinations of observations strengthen belief (though the additive rule is not clear). It also solves the problem of the priors: initially, the vector has zero length – equivalent to no belief in *any* of the hypotheses – and therefore no direction at all! On a linear scale for odds, we have the advantage that each axis is simply counting: to combine new data we simply add it, and the vectors add. But if we used a log scale, then likelihoods would obey ordinary vector summation (the support vector), but unfortunately the direction would no longer have an obvious meaning.

6.3 What Is Randomness?

One should always be a little improbable.
Oscar Wilde, "Phrases and Philosophies for the Use of the Young"(1894)

The *Oxford English Dictionary* defines randomness as '*The quality or state of lacking a pattern or principle of organization; unpredictability*' (Simpson and Weiner 1989). But as we have seen with information, noise, and probability itself, randomness defined in this way is entirely subjective. Some can see the pattern in 1, 1, 2, 3, 5, 8, 13, 21, 34, 55, 89, 144 … because they have come across the Fibonacci series before: others, who haven't, may reasonably think the pattern random. Or suppose, for example, we are told to multiply two n-digit numbers together: what is the nth digit of the answer? For $n = 1$, we learn the answers off by rote at school. But suppose $n = 10$: the answer is just as determinate, but it is unlikely that we already know it. Anything we don't know can be regarded as a random hypothesis (Keynes 1921), for example, '*The number of peanuts in this packet is even.*' It is simply too much trouble to ascertain how the bag-filling machine works. But even a roulette wheel is merely a machine and, if we study it patiently enough, will yield some information about propensity; indeed sufficient is already known to make money from it (Bass 1991).

6.3.1 Benefits of Randomness

Such a system would be a rational decision-maker. But two aspects of it will seem implausible, in that they appear gratuitously to degrade the system's performance. Why have a rise-to-threshold decision mechanism at all, when the information required to make the decision – prior support and log likelihood – is already present at the start of the rise, so that in principle a choice could be made at once? And why introduce the deliberate noise represented by the random variation of slope from trial to trial, which can only increase the incidence of errors?

In fact, both of these features can in fact be seen as advantages. The procrastination introduced by a rise-to-threshold, combined with a random handicap, means that the race is not always to the quickest, and that late-arriving stimuli – whether through weakness or simply as a result of a sudden change in circumstances – have an opportunity to compete against stronger ones. This can be seen, for instance, in the Wheeless task (Section 4.9.2) (Wheeless, Boynton et al. 1966). A subject asked to look at a target that moves to the left, and then – after a pause – moves to the right, will on a random proportion of trials ignore the initial stimulus altogether and simply go straight to the right. The general stochastic properties of such behaviour accord very well with a linear rise-to-threshold model (Noorani and Carpenter 2015), which provides a simple explanation of the observed relationship between the length of time spent by the target on the left, and the probability of the first saccade being made in that direction. As in real life, procrastination allows time in which to consider a number of alternatives, for which not all the evidence may have been present at the moment the choice could first be made (see Section 6.6). In addition, a race in which the winner takes all provides a decisive result, even when the merits of the contenders are evenly matched, and prevents both vacillatory behaviour, inappropriate compromises (as, for instance, making a saccade to a point half-way between two stimuli), or fatal indecision – like Buridan's Ass, starving to death when equidistant from two indistinguishably delicious bundles of hay (Carpenter 1994).

So far, LATER has been presented as a kind of idealised decision-maker. But in one respect it does not seem at all ideal, or even rational: the gratuitous randomness of the rate of rise of the decision signal. The most obvious effect of this randomness is that it makes reaction times unnecessarily variable. If this were all it did, the consequences would not be of great significance: if the timing of our responses differs on different occasions by a few milliseconds, does this matter very much?

If there is only one stimulus on each trial, demanding a single response, then the answer is probably no. But in the world outside the laboratory, there are large numbers of stimuli, and large numbers of possible corresponding responses. One of LATER's virtues is providing a mechanism for choosing between competing hypotheses, by making them run a kind of handicap race: the hypothesis reaching the finishing line first wins and initiates the corresponding response. As we have seen, this provides a mechanism for weighing past experience against present evidence, so that we do not necessarily respond either to those stimuli we most expect, or to those that are too improbable even though they seem to fit the present sense-data. Furthermore, a hypothesis that is very strong in relation to its competitors will be largely unaffected by this randomness: it applies only to those which are more closely matched, when a 'wrong' response is less likely to matter. A consequence of running races to decide the winner is that if there is an element of randomness in the speed of competitors, then there will necessarily be an element of randomness in the final outcome. Not just our timing will be unpredictable: so will our choices.

But what could possibly be the point of deliberately not choosing the best response? It turns out that there are good biological reasons for making our actions at least somewhat random. To see what they are, we need to consider something called game theory.

6.3.2 Game Theory

Game theory flourished during the 1950s, perhaps inspired by the aggressive stand-offs of the Cold War. But the basic concept that randomness can be rational had already been formulated by R. A. Fisher as early as 1934 (Fisher 1934) in the context of card games. In the simplest formal example, two players compete in a 'zero-sum' game: what is won by player A is lost by player B. Each player has just two alternative moves at each turn, and decide their moves secretly and simultaneously, generating an outcome when their decisions are actually revealed. An important result in the analysis of certain kinds of formalised games is that the only winning strategy is to make one's behaviour as unpredictable as possible. A good example is the game we have probably all played as children, in which I secrete a coin in one of my hands and you have to guess which it is. If I always put it in the same hand, then you will eventually realise this and win every time. Similarly, if you always make the same guess, I will eventually win every time. But the same is true in the long term if there is even just the slightest tendency to favour one hand rather than the other. Conversely, you must not guess one side more often than the other, or I will modify my hiding accordingly. It is not difficult to show that the correct strategy, which cannot be beaten, is to be as unpredictably random as possible. On average, each player will then win exactly half the time (Figure 6.4).

This is not a mere mathematical abstraction. There are many real games for which prediction of the opponent's behaviour confers an obvious advantage: think of penalties in soccer, of bowling in cricket, of returning a serve in tennis. It is therefore essential to

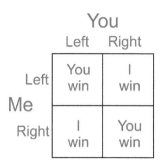

Figure 6.4 A zero-sum game. I hide an object in my left or right hand, you to try to guess which. The optimum strategy for both players is to be as unpredictably random as possible.

be as unpredictable as possible. In penalty shoot-outs, for instance, the shooter is trying hard to prevent the goalie predicting which side of the net they are aiming at, while the goalie is trying to make equally unpredictable the direction in which they are going to leap.

Of course, this assumes that the players are solely motivated by the desire to 'win'; but in a more social context altruism and cooperation may also need to be considered (Lee 2008).

And in the real world of predator–prey relationships, whether the classic Chaplinesque chase round the kitchen table or companies trying to outguess each other's take-over manoeuvres, the same drive for unpredictability is obvious. As the lion chases the bounding wildebeest, if the wildebeest jumps to the left when the lion thinks it's going to jump to the right, it may avoid becoming lunch; and the lion who is not equally unpredictable in his movements will go hungry.

In a more general sense, one may also argue that a degree of randomness in response is desirable in itself, both to ensure that over-learning of a stereotyped response does not prevent serendipity, the chance discovery of an even better one that is initially improbable. It is a commonplace of game theory (von Neumann and Morgenstern 1947) that optimum strategies in such games demand a random element in making decisions for action; there is some evidence that neurons in prefrontal cortex may be doing precisely that (Baraclough, Conroy et al. 2004). The biological benefit of randomness in general is also obvious when one considers the process of sexual reproduction (Fisher 1934).

6.3.3 Imagination and Creativity

Or in the night, imagining some fear,
How easy is a bush supposed a bear!
Shakespeare, Midsummer Night's Dream, *V.i (1595)*

Thus, there are very good reasons for making one's actions unpredictable, and they are not just to do with direct predator–prey game-like interactions. If we always responded in exactly the same way to the same set of circumstances, we would never stumble across new, improved ways of doing things. Exploration, discovery, invention, creativity – the whole of science and the arts, in fact – depend on this mechanism of randomness. There are two slightly different ways in which this kind of behaviour can be generated by LATER. One possibility is to have a relatively low input level, resulting in a bigger contribution from past rather than present data. The result will be obsessional, ruminative behaviour, which may nevertheless be novel in extracting aspects of the stored model that have not previously been noticed: what we commonly call 'thinking'. The other mechanism is when the threshold is low, so that relatively 'wacky' decisions are made (as, for instance, by the maverick units underlying early saccades (Chapter 2, Section 2.2). The cortex will then tend to free-wheel, so that deciding on one hypothesis tends to trigger another equally unlikely one: it is not implausible to see here the origin of dreaming, where each episode seems perfectly logical in relation to what has just been experienced. When we are awake, the same mechanism will generate the new responses to stimuli that form the basis of what we normally call explorative, imaginative behaviour that stops us from being stuck in a behavioural groove.

Finally, the most obvious example of randomness and its benefits is the biological creativity that is due ultimately to randomness in the mechanism of reproduction (Fisher 1950).

6.4 Reward and Utility

Choice of action demands consideration of what decision-theorists call *utility*. Utility is the payoff associated with different decisions, while expected utility is a measure of how much utility, on average, we would expect from a particular response. For a given response A, it is simply equal to $p(A) * U(A)$, where $U(A)$ is the intrinsic value of making response A.

As a result, if we calculate the 'best' response solely on the basis of which is most likely, we may find that some other response represents the best decision in terms of expected utility. Take a game show where a contestant must choose one of two boxes, only one of which contains a prize. The prize in the first is highly valuable, in the second is worth much less but less likely to be empty. If its expected utility is higher, then that is the one to go for. Similarly, if a clinical test suggests the possibility of cancer, but it is very much more likely to be something else, the payoff for not carrying out further tests if it is in fact cancer is so much worse than any other outcome that nevertheless one should act not according to the objective probabilities, but in accordance with the expected utilities. Another example is weather prediction, where it is better to predict a hurricane that doesn't happen than fail to predict one that does (Green and Swets 1966).

Clearly, a complete decision mechanism should include consideration of utility – what psychologists call reward or motivation. Since expected utility is what matters, this implies that the decision signals should be scaled in some way to reflect the associated expected utilities. It is not hypotheses that are being decided between here, but actions. Whatever we decide to do, we clearly do not want our perceptions of the world itself to be influenced by what we would like to happen – although of course very often this is what happens in practice, manifested either as wishful thinking, or its opposite, paranoia.

So although rational behaviour is undeniably founded on expected utility (Good 1952), this may not have much to do with truth. Since the only purpose of perception is decision and action, the establishment of 'truth' as a middle term is a waste of time. But this might not be true of future decisions. One might argue that one should store information about what we have experienced even though at that time it is of no motivational interest, because in future it might have a positive or a negative utility associated with it. In other words, 'truth' is the bit that doesn't change. Or to put it another way, if we can recall sense-data we could use it subsequently to test hypotheses that were not originally around when the data were originally sensed. The snag is that this will take a lot of storage. Further, utility changes when need changes. Depending on whether we are hungry or thirsty, the utility of a sandwich may be higher or lower than that of a glass of beer. This implies a third level of storage, perhaps motivational maps (Gould and White 1974, Wiener, Paul et al. 1989).

Since rational choices must in the end be based on the product of utility and probability (i.e., expected utility) one might think that the decision signal would be simply displaced – that is, multiplied by the utility (since it's a log scale). But then the prior would also behave like that, and the two together might trigger action through mere excess of greed before there was any evidence for the stimulus at all! But recordings from the caudate nucleus seems to suggest a change of slope of the decision signal (Lauwereyns, Watanabe et al. 2002, Lauwereyns 2010), if this represents an alteration in gain of some subcortical loop that might make anatomical (though perhaps not mathematical) sense.

We still know very little about how the motivational systems of the brain actually work. What is clear is that the basal ganglia play an important part as an interface between the limbic system, whose function is to evaluate stimuli by relating them to primary physiological variables sensed by such structures as the hypothalamus, and to the higher efferent pathways for movement control. We have already seen that an important descending route from cortical saccadic areas to the brainstem is via parts of the basal ganglia, including the caudate nucleus and substantia nigra. At this level, different degrees of motivation do indeed modulate the rate of rise of build-up in the prelude to saccadic initiation (Lauwereyns, Takikawa et al. 2002, Lauwereyns, Watanabe et al. 2002), and human subjects respond faster to targets of high expected value (Milstein and Dorris 2007).

6.4.1 Information as Intrinsic Reward

While it is natural to think of 'reward' in terms of food, drink, or sex, or of course money, which can be exchanged for all three, nevertheless it is worth asking whether there is not something even more fundamental that motivates making saccades in the first place. None of those conventional motivators is directly facilitated by saccades (with the possible exception of leers and winks). So, what is the primary reason for making saccades at all? The answer is that they provide information, foraging the outside world and contributing ceaselessly to that store of information that we call our internal model of the world, which forms the basis of our perceptions and – more importantly – our decisions and actions. It is not difficult to devise experiments that show that reaction time is substantially shortened when the target provides useful information, compared with when it doesn't. It is perhaps surprising that the effect of increasing the amount of information gained appears to cause a self-parallel shifting of the distribution, as would be expected from increasing the overall rate of information supply, rather than the swivel – representing an increase in expected utility – that might have been expected (Figure 6.5).

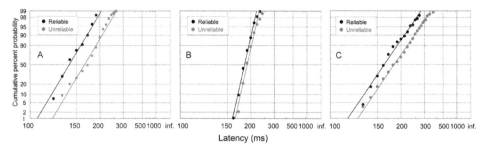

Figure 6.5 Informative targets generate shorter latencies than uninformative ones. Distributions from three subjects presented either with targets that were reliable (always correctly predicting the position of a final target) or unreliable in that sometimes they provided incorrect information (Hänzi, Copley et al. 2011, Bray and Carpenter 2015).

6.5 Free Will and Consciousness

... nothing but a kind of machine or automaton; and the Mind which is in us ... may arrange to sit in the brain merely as a spectator of this play which is acted out in the scene of the body.
William Croone, De ratione motus musculorum *(1667)*

People tend to have strong prejudices about what they consider 'voluntary' rather than 'reflex' actions. But is this actually a helpful distinction? Words like 'mind', 'voluntary', 'reflex', 'attention' are essentially meaningless, adding nothing to our understanding of the brain mechanisms and hinging on what we consider to be 'willed', which is a matter of what we feel about the action at the time. It is not reflected in anything that can be measured in the behaviour itself. Nor is the sense of 'willing' quite as clear-cut as it might at first appear. Holding a conversation, for instance, is something that most people would assume to be 'voluntary'. Yet a moment's reflection shows that normally we do not think about what we are saying before we say it. In ordinary speech, words are uttered before rather than after any consciousness of what has been said: we do indeed know what we think when we hear what we say.

Hence our illusion is that we have 'free will'. What makes us regard some of our actions as 'willed', or voluntary? We call them 'voluntary' when we've seen the decision evolving, 'involuntary' when we haven't: our actions do not seem unpredictable to ourselves because we see them coming to fruition. Indeed, it is this prior knowledge of our own actions that enables us to distinguish between our finger moving as the result of a decision to move it, and because someone has electrically stimulated our ulnar nerve. But being aware, between the decision and the resultant action, of what one is about to do is not at all the same thing as actually willing the movement in the first place. The phenomenon of the (Kornhuber and Deecke 1965) *Bereitschaftspotential* and the related experiments by Libet (Libet, Wright et al. 1979, Libet 1985, Libet, Peall et al. 1991) demonstrate that neural activity starts to build up hundreds of milliseconds before we think we have decided on an action (Chapte5, Figure 5.2).

Take, for instance, sight-reading at the piano – a highly demanding task that on the face of it ought to be entirely conscious and 'voluntary'. Yet any pianist knows that if someone comes up while one is sight-reading it is perfectly possible to have a conversation with them while one's brain and hands are getting on all by themselves with converting the retinal image of the score into appropriate finger movements. Kubie has gone so far as to assert that there is nothing we can do consciously that we cannot also do unconsciously (Kubie 1954).

> *Our present knowledge does not permit us to speak with any show of truth about the more complicated functions of the mind ... hypotheses of this kind have in great numbers reigned in the writings of physiologists from all time. But all of them alike have been feeble, fleeting, and of short life.*
>
> Albrecht von Haller, *Elementa physiologiae corporis humani* (1757)

> *Psychologists ... have a simple faith that experiments will always help them when in fact their puzzles are often due to conceptual muddles.*
>
> J. J. C. Smart, 'Metaphysics, Logic and Theology', in *New Essays in Philosophical Theology*, ed. Antony Flew and Alasdair MacIntyre (1955)

> *They are ill discoverers that think there is no land, when they can see nothing but sea.*
>
> Francis Bacon, *The Advancement of Learning* (1605)

Are we just machines? I want to start with a rather intriguing idea. It's from a 1940s textbook: a genre of illustration common at the time, designed to encourage students to think of Man as a piece of equipment, *l'homme machine* .... A ghost thrusts in from another universe that throws a switch that starts the current flowing and all the gears turning – a complete cop-out for describing how the brain may work! This epitomises the way in which people were perfectly happy with physiological machinery *below* the neck, but *above* it their nerve fails.

Can we justify making a distinction between the body and the brain? One thing we can agree on is that the brain's function is to convert patterns of sensory input into patterns of motor outputs, using billions of neurons that gradually transform these patterns from level to level – an entirely mechanical and automatic process.

Most people find this deeply disturbing: if the brain's a *thing*, does that mean *we* are things too?

> *The idea that my sucker is moving through thought itself, through emotion and reason, that memories, dreams and reflections should simply consist of jelly, is simply too strange to understand.*
>
> Henry Marsh, neurosurgeon. *Guardian*, 15 November 2014

So, they reject the idea that it is a machine and start making metaphysical noises: that there is some kind of soul or mind or spirit, that it's this that makes them do things.

What we all feel in fact – let's be honest – is something more like Figure 6.6: sometimes called the *little man in the head* – another shockingly *explicit* illustration. There is the little man, looking at the screen and apparently playing a sort of cerebral Hammond organ. A *natural* way to look at it, but perhaps not a very *satisfying* one from intellectual point of view, not least because it obviously prompts the question of whether the little man has a little man in *his* head!

Historically, there has been an ongoing struggle between these two conceptions, mind and matter. Originally spirit was in the ascendant: an obvious feature of the brain is the pair of large ventricles, hollow chambers filled with fluid. This fluid was felt to be much more than just *physical* liquid: mysterious vital spirit that actually caused things to happen (Figure 6.7). There was a clear interface: consciousness, volition, mind.

But with the coming of a new mechanical rationalism in the seventeenth century this view began to be modified, these mysterious fluids began to be thought of rather less

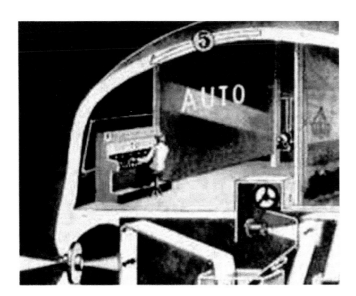

Figure 6.6 Little man in head. He recognises 'auto' and makes an appropriate response.

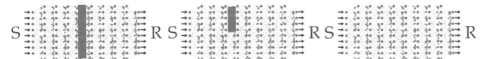

Figure 6.7 Early understanding suggested a barrier that forced all stimuli to act via the 'spirit'; later, it recognised that some responses could by-pass the barrier as part of the 'machinery' of the brain; finally, all actions were assumed to be the consequence of a purely metaphysical process.

spiritually and more prosaically as *physical* fluids, like the water in the complex hydraulic systems then all the rage, for instance, at Versailles. Descartes described what he called the 'reasoning soul' as controlling the flow to the muscles as the *fontenier* controls the water pressure in the royal gardens:

> *You may have seen in the grottoes and fountains in our royal gardens that the simple force of the water is sufficient to power various machines, and even to set various instruments playing, or make them pronounce words. Indeed, one may very well compare the nerves of the body with the tubes of these fountains, the muscles and tendons with the other diverse engines and springs which serve to move these machines, and the Animal Spirits, whose reservoirs are the ventricles, with the water that puts them into motion.*

Descartes, *Discours de la méthode* (1656)

Talking in the broadest possible terms, what we have seen historically is a sort of struggle between these two conceptions, between mind and matter: it is curious how throughout the ages the machinery part of the brain has almost always been conceived in terms of the latest modish technology of the period.

Though the 'spiritual' part was banished from the ventricles, Descartes thought it still had an essential role, but concentrated in just one tiny organ at the heart of the brain – the *pineal*. Tiny, but remarkably like the man in the cab of a mechanical digger pulling the *delicate* little levers that control the *powerful flow* of hydraulic fluid. So now the big chunk of spirit in the middle of the brain had **shrunk** down to a tiny sliver, the pineal: *ghost in the machine.*

At about the same time, the Industrial Revolution was making people familiar with machines that seemed to mimic what had been thought to be purely human capabilities: the apparently intelligent self-acting governors on steam engines, the intricate patterns of the automatic Jacquard loom, programmed by punched cards. With the discovery of electricity, people naturally seized on the idea that these fluids were probably electrical. Above all, later, there emerged the development of the telephone exchange – the most complex human-made structures had ever seen, thrillingly massive bundles of cables like nerve fibres, rows and rows of repetitive units like cortical neurons, with the soul somewhat side-lined as the lonely switchboard operator.

And finally, the arrival of the computer, programmed by literally plugging various units together in particular ways. Yet they seemed terrified of suggesting that their machines could actually *think:* and this terror is a recurring theme in the history of the development of the computer?

This fear has been with us a long time. As far back as 1642 Pascal invented one of the first calculating machines, the Pascaline. Now, it may seem perfectly harmless to us, but at the time it caused consternation amongst the public. He felt compelled to write, *The arithmetical machine achieves results which come closer to thought than anything animals do: but it does nothing to make us say that it has volition.* Again, when Babbage designed his pioneering mechanical computer, the Analytical Engine, his groupie/fan Ada Augusta, Countess of Lovelace, wrote in 1842:

> It is desirable to guard against the possibility of exaggerated ideas that might arise as to the powers of the Analytical Engine. The Analytical Engine has no pretensions whatever to originate anything. Its province is to assist us in making available what we are already acquainted with.
>
> Charles Babbage, 'Letter to Sir David Brewster, LLD.,
> On the Subject of Mr. Babbage's Calculating Engines'

Throughout the eighteenth and nineteenth centuries there was a vogue for exhibitions of ever more realistic mechanical automata attracting huge crowds of visitors – some rather silly, some more sophisticated, like Winkel's Componium, that actually composed music, or my absolute favourite, John Clark's Eureka of 1845 that generated Latin hexameters: not only clever, but splendidly patriotic.

> Each verse remains stationary and visible a sufficient time for a copy of it to be taken; it may be made to go on continually, producing in one day and night, or twenty-four hours, about 1440 Latin verses. During the composition of each line, a cylinder in the interior of the machine performs the National Anthem.
>
> 'An Extraordinary Typewriter', *Illustrated London News*, 8 November 1856

Then the delicious, creepy thrill people seemed to get from robots in the early twentieth century; but even if it were true that everything the brain does could be done by a machine, does not of course follow that the brain *itself* must be a machine. It was obvious that a great deal of our behaviour really doesn't go through the 'spirit' bit at all. Furthermore, electrical stimulation of the surface of the brain revealed orderly machine-like maps like this one of the dog by Ferrier in 1886, giving rise to the pseudo-science of phrenology; all the different bits of the brain seemed to be wired up to each other. The brain was simply a kind of telephone exchange. Everything suddenly seemed terribly clear, 'pathways' joining 'centres' for this that were thought to explain everything.

So, is that it? Has metaphysics been squeezed out altogether? Must we finally concede that we are indeed just machines?

There is still one refuge for those still uncomfortable with this conclusion. A characteristic of machines is that on the whole they are rather predictable – their behaviour more or less determined by the instructions we give them – whereas people are not. Indeed, as soon as a machine starts behaving unpredictably, what do we say? '*It has a mind of its own.*' Unlike the machine, we have – or *appear* to have – free will.

So – slightly absurdly – we turn the argument on its head: instead of saying we cannot be machines because we can *think* and machines can't, which is obviously untrue, we now argue the opposite: we cannot be machines because we can act *irrationally* and machines can't. Unfortunately, this won't do either.

In the end, we come back to how it feels: the little man in the head. Most of my scientific colleagues think one should just *ignore* how it feels, ignore everything not based on objective scientific fact. I don't agree with them, and I want to finish by presenting one way in which it is possible to reconcile the metaphysical with the physical: the idea that everything we do is determined by the machinery in our heads with the sense we clearly all have of our own conscious perception of the world. It is simply, in effect, to allow that what we feel is the literal truth: that there *is* a metaphysical entity of some kind whose nature is entirely beyond the probing of science, capable of monitoring much (but not all) of what goes on in the brain and giving rise to consciousness. Note that this is perfectly compatible with the ordinary laws of physics such as the law of conservation of energy. The official name for such a view is 'epiphenomenalism', but I prefer to think of it as *one-way Cartesianism*: The other way is the idea of volition, which I think has to be ruled out on scientific grounds, not least because it violates conservation of energy, and in any case is a hypothesis we have no need of – the most complex tasks we do consciously, for example, playing the piano – can in fact be done equally well unconsciously. In neurophysiological terms, there is no necessity whatever for the ghost in the machine, for anything except an unbroken chain of neurons all the way from sensory receptors to motor neurons. In any case, it is a hypothesis we have no need of – as we have seen, everything the brain does, *can* be explained by neural machinery.

So why do we have the illusion of conscious volition, and the accompanying sense of free will? I think what we mean by a voluntary action – what Wittgenstein characterised as the difference between '*my arm goes up*' and '*I lift my arm*' – is that we are aware of the neural processes that lead to *some* actions – we see them coming – but not *others*, and the former are what we call voluntary. As a matter of fact, if you think critically about which of your actions really are voluntary, you soon begin to see how few of them really are. Clearly, most of what we do is not voluntary – where you placed your feet as you walked into this room – and even very complex things like playing the piano or speaking.

People sometimes object to this formulation on moral grounds: it means you can't *blame* people for things, and certainly not inflict the barbarity of punishing them: do we punish a broken watch? Others complain that it makes the soul pointless, just a passive observer. Personally, I find the idea of the soul as a sort of perpetual tourist, carried round by our bodies and enjoying the drama of daily life, quite attractive. The moral is clear: *enjoy your trip!*

The brain is what makes the subjective objective: so, instead of 'subjective! Shock horror!!!' we have 'How would you design a machine to form judgments about probabilities on the basis of the information that it has actually received?'

Here is a trick for getting out of lazy habits about free will: instead of saying 'I think' say ' Roger thinks' or 'Roger's brain thinks'; instead of 'I stole the book' use ' Roger stole the book' or 'Roger's brain stole the book'.

There was undoubtedly a growing conviction that a machine *could* do much – maybe everything – that a human brain was capable of. But in strict logical terms, being able to demonstrate that a machine can do things the brain does, does *not* of course prove that the brain itself must therefore be a machine. That requires *physiological experiments*.

> *I removed the two cerebral lobes from a healthy chicken. I had scarcely removed the brain before the sight of both eyes was suddenly lost; the hearing was also gone and the animal did not give the slightest sign of volition, but kept itself perfectly upright upon its legs, and walked when it was stimulated – or when it was pushed. When thrown into the air, it flew; and swallowed water when it was put into its beak. The animal, thus deprived of its cerebrum, survived ten whole months in a state of perfect health.*
>
> Jean Flourens, *Encyclopedia Britannica* (1911)

So, it seemed that a great deal of our behaviour really didn't have to go through the 'spirit' bit at all. And even the higher areas seemed to be organised in a systematic, machine-like way, just like the telephone exchanges: electrical stimulation of the surface of the brain revealed orderly maps like the one of the dog by Ferrier (1886). So, by about 1900 the frontiers had been firmly pushed back. Everything suddenly seemed terribly clear: programmable pathways joining 'centres' for this and that were thought to explain everything – reminiscent of the much earlier pseudo-science of phrenology, and looking forward to the similar excesses of magnetic resonance brain imaging.

So, is that it? Has metaphysics been squeezed out altogether? Are we indeed just machines? Scary . . .

Is it possible to reconcile these two things, that our actions are indeed produced by a neural machine, but that there is something metaphysical as well? Start by having a closer look at the actual brain, rather than metaphors of the brain, and our current understanding of how it actually works.

In fact, looking at the brain is not tremendously helpful, as its appearance gives very little away about *what it does*, let alone *how it works*. If you look at the heart, for instance, particularly in the living animal, its function is pretty obvious: it's full of tubes and valves. But open up the skull: what do we see? A rather repulsive lump of fibrous porridge. No wonder some early natural philosophers were so completely at sea about what it did: Aristotle believed that the brain's function was to cool the blood, rather like a car's radiator.

The fibrous porridge is actually made up of cells called neurons. A neuron is a device for gathering and disseminating information by giving and receiving contacts with many other neurons. Much of the pioneering work on how neurons work together in an integrated way is due to Sir Charles Sherrington.

So, we can represent the brain in a rather abstract way, something like this: each neuron is a computer in its own right, and the reason we're so clever is that we have such an extraordinary number of these computers acting together in parallel. And that's really all you need to know to understand how the brain works. The proof is that human-made neural networks, implemented in tiny computers like the one in your smartphone, can do some remarkably intelligent things, recognising handwriting or speech, even though their constituent units are far stupider than neurons, and there are a lot less of them.

So, to summarise the position so far, it seems on the one hand that machines are capable of doing everything that the brain does, and on the other hand that the brain itself does indeed function purely mechanistically. However, there is still one refuge for those who find this conclusion distasteful. Unlike the machine, we have – or *appear* to have – free will.

One might perhaps have thought that the existence of roulette wheels was evidence against this, but it isn't, since it can be argued that roulette wheels are perfectly determined – with enough information, we can calculate where the ball is going to land. More relevant are recent experiments that seem to suggest that our unpredictability and the accompanying sense of free will are in fact due to a deliberate process of neural randomisation, a specific neural mechanism within the brain whose function is, as it were, to weave *a degree of surprise* into our actions. Because the world is full of things, randomness of timing creates randomness of choice.

> ... *nothing but a kind of machine or automaton; and the Mind which is in us ... may arrange to sit in the brain merely as a spectator of this play which is acted out in the scene of the body.*
> William Croone, *De ratione motus musculorum* (1664)

Finally, towards the end of *War and Peace*, Tolstoy wrote:

> *During the whole of that period, Napoleon, who seems to us to have been the leader of all those movements – as the figurehead of a ship may seem to a savage to guide the vessel – acted like a child who, holding a couple of strings inside a carriage, thinks he is driving it.*
> Tolstoy, *War and Peace*, Book XIII, Chapter X (1869)

> ... *We in our skulls are like the child in the carriage.*
> *We are like stones rolling downhill but asserting violently that we choose to do so.*
> Baruch Spinoza, *Ethics* (1993/1677)

6.6 Probability: The Language of the Brain

All knowledge degenerates into probability
David Hume, A Treatise of Human Nature *(1739)*

We think we perceive exactly what goes on around us, but what we are actually doing is guessing – forming hypotheses – about the objects around us on the basis of the rather limited evidence coming from our senses. Meanwhile, we are building up this virtual model in our heads on the basis of associations. Our perceptions are based much more on this model than on actual incoming sensory information. Our eyes are perpetually moving about, filling in details in the model of what's around us. We shut our eyes and it's all still there.

So, perception is dominated by our prior probabilities, our expectations about the world, which depend on the circumstances – circumstantial evidence, in fact. We recognise someone coming down the street partly because we use fragments of visual information about their appearance, but also a host of background information about how likely it is that they are in fact there at this particular time of day. Often, we fail to recognise someone we know very well because it's an unfamiliar place – perhaps abroad – and the context makes it seem unlikely that they are there. Anyone who had to do proof-reading knows how difficult it is to see what is actually there rather than simply predictable from the context. As Bartlett (1932, p. 82) has put it: '*The almost inevitable*

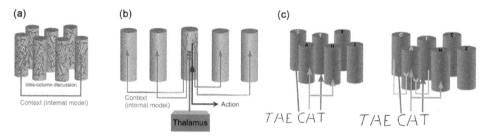

Figure 6.8 Columns as committees. (a) Most neurons in a cortical column talk to each other, sharing their information (red). (b) An internal model is built up, using the context provided other columns by associational fibres (blue). (c) An example: the 'A' in 'THE CAT' is ambiguous (pink) – it could be an 'A' or an'H' – but the internal model – driven by 'C' and 'T' – favours 'A'.

impulse is to visualize a few letters and thence to infer the whole word, and even from part of a sentence to infer the rest and it requires a strong and persistent effort to insist that the eye shall not thus shirk its work of adequate observation and it requires a strong and persistent effort to insist that the eye shall not thus shirk its work of adequate observation.' Conversely, one may briefly perceive events which the context makes irresistibly likely. *'It happened in my own experience that someone turned on the wireless and saw the dial light up for a moment and then go out. Inspection showed that the wireless was disconnected from the mains and could not have lit up at all'* (Tyrrell 1946). The structure of the cerebral cortex is ideally suited to generating associations of this kind – in fact, it is why it evolved in the first place. Cortex is arranged as columns of neurons that interact with one another and form an internal model of the outside world (Figure 6.8). We can think of this internal model of the world as a huge network of interacting conditional probabilities, embodied as plastic synapses with variable strengths.

6.6.1 Interpreting Neural Networks

Log likelihood is the most efficient way of organising a network for inference, for much the same reasons as for detecting stimuli. It is in the language of log likelihood ratios and log odds that the neural implementation of decisions about the existence of hypotheses and about actions to be taken must be expressed (Anderson 1993).

An information theorist would immediately recognise here a situation in which the flow of 'information' from the environment is limited by a noisy channel of communication, one that garbles its messages even when the stimulus itself is essentially free from noise; but the theorist would have little to say about the decision-process itself.

A statistician, on the other hand, would see the analogy with sequential testing. Starting with prior probabilities $p(H_i)$ over the set of hypotheses H (Aantaa, Riekkinen et al. 1973), the data from the sense-organ could be considered as a series of fragments of evidence E. Then we can make revised estimates $p'(H_i)$ from past experience of $p(E|H_i)$ (Figure 6.9). These estimates will increase or decrease with time as more evidence is accumulated, more or less rapidly as the noise level is lower or higher, until one of them reaches a threshold that represents some notional level of 'significance' (see Appendix 1, App 1.8.4).

And the neurophysiologist will naturally be inclined to think more prosaically in terms of neurons that respond to stimuli by generating noisy signals, and which may summate in space or time to generate decisions that are less noisy than the signals that prompt them.

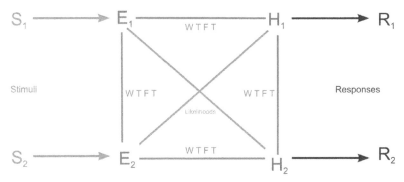

Figure 6.9 Lack of distinction between neurons ultimately driven by *stimuli1* (E_1 and E_2) and those generating *responses* (H_1 and H_2); the learning mechanisms for forming associations between each ('WTFT – Wire Together Fire Together) are the same for E_1, E_2, H_1, and H_2, so that they are all ultimately Hebbian. Note: 'Hebbian' refers to a principle in neuroscience known as Hebb's rule, which states that when two neurons are repeatedly activated at the same time, the connection between them is strengthened.

The foregoing represent three viewpoints, but evidently only a single system. Can a common discourse be found that will link all three? Experience shows that neurophysiologists are adaptable creatures who are happy to incorporate into their models whatever conceptual framework seems most appropriate (or most fashionable). The real difficulty here stems from the theoreticians, the informationists, and the statisticians. Information theory and the principles of statistical inference have never been brought very satisfactorily into line with one another, perhaps because a situation has never arisen where they have been forced to pull in harness because they are both self-evidently talking about the same thing. Here in the brain, we have a piece of neuronal hardware that is actually doing statistical inference, and actually exhibiting the kinds of channel-like behaviour that information theory has always talked about.

The fundamental link between the three areas is of course the idea that the perceived likelihood of a hypothesis changes as the result of information that is received. But it is in only a few cases – perhaps rather artificial ones – that likelihood can be assigned the same kind of precise objective meaning that 'probability' can. This immediately introduces a psychological element into the discussion, something whose unmathematical qualities have undoubtedly led to much of the confusion and dispute that this whole area has engendered amongst both information theorists and statisticians. But it need not do so, for 'hypothesis' of course implies a brain in which the hypothesis is embedded quite literally and physically, and 'likelihood' equally implies the existence of some physical variable associated with that hypothesis.

A statistician may feel some delicacy about the propriety of putting a number to the prior probability of a hypothesis – whether God exists, to take an extreme (but no doubt important) example – but our own neurons are not so squeamish; whatever we feel about some particular hypothesis has its exact physical counterpart in the firing frequency of a neuron or the strength of its synapses. And these physical attributes are the same, whether we are considering a situation where it is legitimate to talk about probabilities of hypotheses (for example, where one has to guess whether a given sample was taken from one urn or another, chosen by tossing a coin) or cases like the theological one where it is not. By facing firmly up to that bug-bear of mind rather than running away from it, by attempting to incorporate its own machinery within a framework that embraces both information and statistical theory, one may hope to avoid some of the unease engendered by purely theoretical approaches.

I would earnestly warn you against trying to find out the reason and explanation of everything. To try and find out the reason for everything is very dangerous and leads to nothing but disappointment and dissatisfaction, unsettling your mind and in the end making you miserable.
Queen Victoria, in a letter to her granddaughter (1883)

Appendix 1 Mathematical

Mathematics is the art of giving the same name to different things.
Henri Poincaré, Science et méthode *(1908)*

For those who appreciate such things, this Appendix brings together the more purely mathematical aspects of what has been discussed in the preceding chapters.

App 1.1 Notation

App 1.1.1 General

t	Time
s	Reciprocal time, or promptness
i	trial index
s_i	Reciprocal latency: set of promptnesses
N	Number of trials
T, T_i	Latency, set of latencies
T_M	Median latency
$L(t)$	Probability density function for latency
$R(s)$	Probability density function for reciprocal latency
$C(s)$	Cumulative frequency of s_i
$C(0)$	Terminal frequency of s_i
$P(x)$	Cumulative normal function
$Q(x)$	Complement of the cumulative normal function: $Q = (1 - P)$
S	Decision signal
S_0	Initial value of S
S_T	Threshold value of S that initiates a response
θ	Range of S: $(S_T - S_0)$
r, r_i	Rate of rise of S, set of rates of rise
μ	Median of r_i
σ^2	Variance of r_i
δ	Delay
τ	Time constant
$E(x)$	Expected value of x

App 1.1.2 Specific Terminology for Inference

In addition to probability itself, there are many subsidiary concepts that need to be name and defined. The following does not claim to be exhaustive: for a more complete list, covering standard notation in information theory, see Good (1955). It is unfortunate that different authors have often introduced new names for entities that already existed.

|	given	
:	provided by	
'	modified by observation	
,	list separator for propositions	
X, Y, A, B, etc.	propositions	
H	hypothetical proposition	
~H	Negation of H	
$H_1, H_2, H_3, \ldots$	Composite hypothesis	
E	event	
p, q	probabilities	
odds(A,B)		$p(A)/p(B)$
lod(A,B)	Log odds	$\log(p(A)/p(B))$
ent(H)	expected information concerning H	E I(H)
ent(p)	total expected information	$-p \log(p) - (1 - p)\log(1 - p)$
ent(H:E$_j$)	entropy concerning H provided by E$_j$	$E_j \Sigma_i\, p(H_i|E_j)I(H_i:E_j)$.

In Shannon terms:

ent (H:E)	Rate of transmission, R	
$H(x)$	ent(H)	
$H(x,y)$	ent(H.E)	
$H_x(y)$	ent(E|H)	
$H_y(x)$	ent(H|E)	
Expectation of ent (H:Ej) before Ej observed	$\Sigma_j\, p(E_j)$ ent $(H{:}E_j)$ = ent (E:H)	

ev(H:E)	Experimental support	sur(E|~
I(H:E)	support	log(p(E|H)/p(E))
I(H$_i$:E)	composite support	log(p(E|H$_i$)/p(E)) = log(p(E|H$_i$)/ $\Sigma_j\,(p$(E|H$_j$)p(H$_j$))
cred'(H)	ev(H:E) + cred(H)	
U(X)	impossibility	U(X) = 1/p (X)

same as Jeffreys' improbability, imp(X) = 1/p(X) (Jeffreys 1931)

$-\log(p$ (X) identical with (Good 1955, Good 1971) Good's I(X)

W(H$_1$, H$_2$: E)	weight of evidence concerning (H$_1$ v. H$_2$) provided by E

log(p(E\|H$_1$)/p(E\|H$_2$) = I(H$_1$: E) – I(H$_2$:E)

Information I = $_p\int^1$ (1/x)dx, = $-\log(p)$

('work' done in moving from one probability to another, realised when found true).

bel	bel as the only measure of probability (the most fundamental)
likelihood	p(E|H)
likelihood ratio	p(E|H)/p(E|~H)

support	log likelihood ratio (LLR)	log(p(E|H)/p(E|~H)) or I(E|H) – I(E|~H)
support	I(H:E)	log (p (E|H)/p (E))

Belief increases linearly in a series of identical trials with identical outcomes (the support is constant). In a strict Peircean formulation, ~H is tricky, because there may be no corresponding p(E); but provided there is a set of actual alternative hypotheses to choose from, neural implementation is not a problem

So (I' – I) or log(p/p') is a measure of information gained or lost through experience, per axis.

sex(p)	(Weaver 1948) surprise index	$\mathscr{E}\,(\sim p)/p$: (expected $\sim p$ divided by p actually observed.
	In logarithmic form, $\mathscr{E}$ (log p) – log p	amount of info in event, less the expected amount.

Rational support for A vs. B	I(E|A) – I(E|B)	- this is Edwards' 'support'
Global support for A	I(E|A) – I(E)	- same as corroboration, above
Peirce support for A	I(E|A) – I(E|~A)	- same as confirmation, above, or weight of evidence

The ranges of the some of these functions are:

p	0 to 1
U	1 to ∞
bel	$-\infty$ to $+\infty$

imp   1 to ∞

ent(0)   ent(0) = ent(1) = 0; ent(0.5) = 0.5;
ent(0.25) = 0.5.

App 1.2 Properties of the Recinormal Distribution

In general, a normal distribution is described by the frequency or probability density function, $P(x)$:

$$P(x) = \frac{1}{\sqrt{2\pi}\sigma} e^{-\frac{(x-\mu)^2}{2\sigma^2}}, \qquad \text{(App 1.1)}$$

where μ is the mean of the distribution and σ^2 is the variance (σ is then the standard deviation, a measure of the overall width); μ is also the median value of x, since the distribution is symmetrical: $P(x - \mu) \equiv P(\mu - x)$ for all x.

Corresponding to this probability density function or PDF is the cumulative distribution function or CDF, which is given by:

$$C(x) = \frac{1}{\sqrt{2\pi}\sigma} \int_{-\infty}^{x} e^{-\frac{(z-\mu)^2}{2\sigma^2}} dz. \qquad \text{(App 1.2)}$$

This is S-shaped (Figure App 1.1) and is normalised in the sense that it ranges from 0 to 1.

In a recinormal distribution, the reciprocal of the variate is normally distributed. In the case of reaction times, this means that the probability of a response in a particular trial having a latency T whose reciprocal $(S = 1/T)$ lies between s and $s + ds$ is:

$$R(s) = \frac{-1}{\sigma\sqrt{2\pi}} e^{-\frac{(s-\mu)^2}{2\sigma^2}} ds, \qquad \text{(App 1.3)}$$

where the mean (and also median) of the distribution is μ and σ^2 is the variance.

From this the probability density of the set of original reaction times we can derive T_i as

$$L(t) = \frac{1}{t^2\sigma\sqrt{2\pi}} e^{-\frac{(1-\mu t)^2}{2t^2\sigma^2}} dt. \qquad \text{(App 1.4)}$$

This is a positively skewed distribution whose median value T_M, is $1/\mu$, but whose mean and variance do not have simple analytical forms.

Typical plots of $R(s)$ and $L(t)$ are shown in Figure App 1.2. When plotting reciprocal latencies, it is helpful to have the origin $(s = 0)$ on the right rather than the left, so that latencies still increase to the right. It also aids comprehension to use a non-linear (reciprocal) scale of

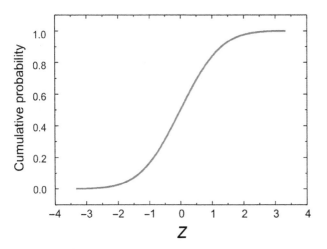

Figure App 1.1 $C(X)$, plotted cumulatively. Z is in units of standard deviation, σ.

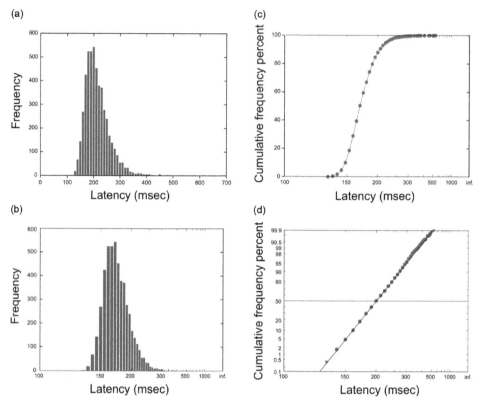

Figure App 1.2 (a,b) Frequency histograms of a simulated recinormal distribution ($N = 5000$, $\mu = 5$, $\sigma = 1$), plotting the probability density for the 'raw' latency T (a), and (b), for its reciprocal, S. Note that latency increases to the right in each case. (c,d) Cumulative frequency plots of the same distribution, using a linear ordinate (c), and a probit scale (d: a reciprobit plot), that generates a straight line if the distribution is indeed Gaussian. The line shown was fitted by minimising the Kolmogorov–Smirnov one-sample statistic.

latencies rather than a linear scale of reciprocal latencies.

If the recinormal distribution is obeyed, a straight line will be obtained: if its slope is μ and it intersects the $t = \infty$ axis at an ordinate k, then $\mu = k/\mu$ and $\sigma = 1/\mu$. Such a plot may be called a *reciprobit plot*, and is illustrated in Figure App 1.2(d). Probabilities are marked on the left-hand ordinate, probits on the right; the reciprocal time scale lies along the bottom, from right to left so that time increases to the right. A scale of reciprocal latency or promptness can be added above. Two critical points on the line have well-defined meanings: where it passes through the horizontal 50% line is the median latency,

T_M, while the intercept k represents the probability that no response to the stimulus ever occurs at all. For easily detected stimuli k is typically of the order of 6–9, and the corresponding probability is so small as to be meaningless. But if the detectability of the stimulus is reduced to near threshold, for instance by reducing the contrast if it is visual, k will become a measurable percentage. k is also the ratio μ/σ, so that under a change in time-scale the line simply swivels around the intercept point.

For a normal distribution the standard error of the median is $1.25\ \sigma/\sqrt{N}$ (Kendall and Stuart 1968); applying this to the recinormal distribution, the standard error of the median latency will be given approximately by multiplying it by $1.25/k\sqrt{N}$. Thus, in a typical experiment, with a median latency of 200 ms, $k = 7$, and $N = 400$, the standard error is about 1.7 ms; such a figure can, however, be misleading, since measurements of successive medians of this kind shows them to be more widely scattered than Figure App 1.2 implies. Latency measurements seem to be subject to random fluctuations over long periods of time, with a noise power spectrum that shows some of the characteristics of $1/f$ noise (Gilden, Thornton et al. 1995, Wagenmakers, Farrell et al. 2004); for this reason, it is necessary to pay careful attention to experimental design when trying to compare the effects of different conditions, and to be aware that the standard error calculated for any one run underestimates the variation to be expected between runs.

App 1.3 Models for Latency Distributions

From time to time, but particularly in the 1960s and 1970s, attempts have been made to discover theoretical functions that could be used to describe reaction time distributions. Some have been derived from theoretical considerations, others purely empirically; some have many parameters, others admirably few. The review that follows does not claim to be comprehensive, or to attempt to compare their success in fitting observed data, or to assess their biological plausibility, but simply to provide a gallery illustrating their general characteristics. By plotting the functions as reciprobit plots, it is relatively easy to see in what ways they differ significantly from LATER-like behaviour. The most thorough way to do this would be simply to repeat the fitting of all the data that have been used here with the rival models, and see whether they perform better or worse. But this would have entailed a very great deal of labour, of a rather negative kind. The procedure actually adopted was to take each of the alternative models in turn, and display their distributions as reciprobit plots for different combinations of the parameters. In this way, one can establish combinations of their parameters that give the nearest approximations to particular recinormal distributions, and then run simulations with numbers of trials of the same order of magnitude as are typically used and see whether the results produce statistically acceptable fits. In this way, one can establish which models are at least compatible with the recinormal distribution under ordinary conditions. Obviously, unless a model is analytically identical with a recinormal distribution, as the number of trials increases a point must eventually come where they are statistically incompatible.

App 1.3.1 Counting Models

A general class of model that is intuitively attractive, and can sometimes generate quite realistic distributions, involves counting events that are generated stochastically and that generate a response when the counts reach some kind of criterion (Pike 1973). They give rise to distributions that are closely related to the gamma and beta functions of stochastic theory, and it may be helpful first to summarise the underlying mathematics, with its rather messy notation: The (complete) gamma function is

$$\Gamma(\alpha) = \int_0^\infty x^{\alpha-1} e^{-x} dx. \qquad \text{(App 1.5)}$$

The corresponding incomplete gamma function has two parameters, and is given by

$$\gamma(\alpha, t) = \int_0^t x^{\alpha-1} e^{-x} dx. \qquad \text{(App 1.6)}$$

A related complete integral, with two parameters, is the complete beta function:

$$B(\alpha, \beta) = \int_0^1 x^{\alpha-1}(1-x)^{\beta-1}dx.$$

(App 1.7)

This in turn has a corresponding incomplete beta function:

$$B_t(\alpha, \beta) = \int_0^t x^{\alpha-1}(1-x)^{\beta-1}dx.$$

(App 1.8)

A useful variant is to consider the incomplete function as a fraction of the whole:

$$I_t(\alpha, \beta) = B_t(\alpha, \beta)/B(\alpha, \beta) \qquad \text{(App 1.9)}$$

The beta-prime function, is derived from I_t:

$$\beta'(t; \alpha, \beta) = I_{\left(\frac{t}{1+t}\right)}(\alpha, \beta). \qquad \text{(App 1.10)}$$

Finally, the CDF of the gamma distribution (not to be confused with the gamma function of which it is a fractional form) is

$$C(t) = \gamma(\alpha, t)/\Gamma(\alpha) \qquad \text{(App 1.11)}$$

A general-purpose class of model, consisting of a number N of gamma-like stages in series, has sometimes been advocated (Lee and Luce 1956, Luce 1960, McGill and Gibbon 1965). Potentially, it could have a vast number of parameters, since each of the N stages could be different, and could be tweaked around to fit almost anything. A simplification (Restle 1961) is to assume each stage to be an identical single decision mechanism with the same exponential form ($\tau = 1/\alpha$); the three parameters are N, α, and a transport delay, δ: the PDF (neglecting δ) is then a gamma function:

$$P(t) = \frac{\alpha^N t^{N-1}}{(N-1)!}e^{-\alpha t}dt. \qquad \text{(App 1.12)}$$

By manipulation of these parameters, one can achieve distributions that look quite straight on a reciprobit plot, at least for the middle and early sections (Figure App 1.3), and only fail the K-S test with extremely large data sets.

App 1.3.2 La Berge Distribution

The simplest counting model is the La Berge model (La Berge 1962). It is based on the idea of sequential sampling at a fixed rate, with a response occurring when a specified number r of samples meets some criterion. The probability of a sample meeting the criterion, given the stimulus, is p, and k samples are made per unit time. The average frequency of responses will then be pk/r. Given that there are only two parameters, the correspondence to a LATER model with a main and early component is generally good (Figure App 1.4), with statistically acceptable fits for $N = 1000$. Potentially it would provide an alternative to the recinormal distribution with an early component, and its theoretical basis is one that lends itself to neurophysiological interpretation, for example in terms of action-potential counting.

App 1.3.3 Van den Berg Model

A further refinement, mentioned earlier, is to envisage that a trial may sometimes result in failure rather than success. Van den Berg's model is in effect a race between successes and failures, whose probabilities per trial (occurring at rate k) are respectively p_s and p_f. If the accumulated number of successes reaches a count of r_p before the count of failures reaches a different criterion, r_f, then a response is made; otherwise, the unit goes into a stop mode, and no response is made at all. It is capable of producing realistic distributions, especially of those observed during spontaneous viewing, though unsatisfactorily steep at long latencies (Figure App 1.5). But it has an intrinsically large number of parameters,

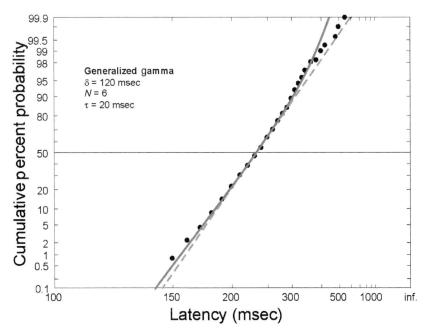

Figure App 1.3 Generalised gamma distribution, with the parameters shown. The red line is the theoretical distribution; the black points show the results of a simulation with 1000 trials, which generated a significance level of $p = 0.85$ (K-S1). The grey dashed line shows the recinormal with the best fit to the theoretical distribution.

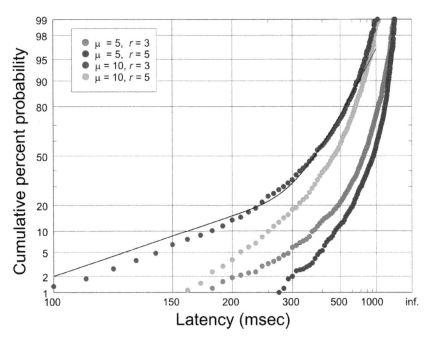

Fig. App 1.4 La Berge distributions (simulations of 1000 trials each) for the values of the parameters shown. The solid line shows a best-fit LATER distribution (with early component) to the distribution for ($\mu = 10$, $r = 3$).

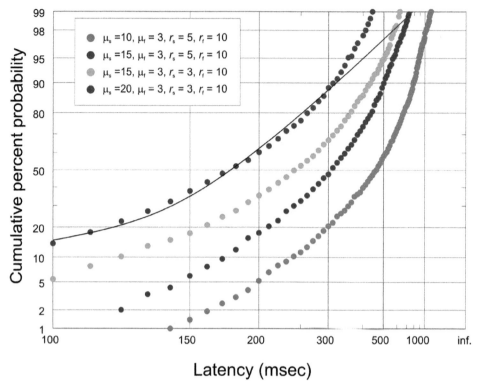

Figure App 1.5 Van den Berg model distributions (simulations of 1000 trials each) for the values of the parameters shown. The black line shows a best-fit LATER distribution (with early component) to the distribution for ($\mu_s = 20$, $\mu_f = 3$, $r_s = 3$, $r_f = 10$).

and of course in spontaneous viewing it is inconceivable that no subsequent saccade would be made at all, as implied by its stop behaviour.

App 1.3.4 Difference Counting

A variation of van den Berg that gets round that last difficulty is to envisage not a draconian stop mechanism as result of accumulated failures, but rather that a running count is kept in which each success adds one and each failure subtracts one: a response is made when the accumulated total reaches a criterion count r. As well as ensuring that some kind of response is made in spontaneous viewing, this model also has one less free parameter, and can produce good fits to spontaneous reaction-time distributions (Figure App 1.6).

App 1.4 Pragmatic Functions

Sometimes it is convenient to use a function that is not based on any particular model, but provides a set of parameters that summarise a distribution in an empirical way. However, the lack of a functional interpretation is a severe drawback.

App 1.4.1 Normex

This consists of a normal distribution convoluted with an exponential (Christie and Luce 1956, Hohle 1965). It requires three parameters, a characteristic time τ, and two dimensionless parameters, α and β, that determine the relative widths of the exponential and Gaussian components respectively. Figure App 1.7 shows reciprobit plots of the Normex distribution for various

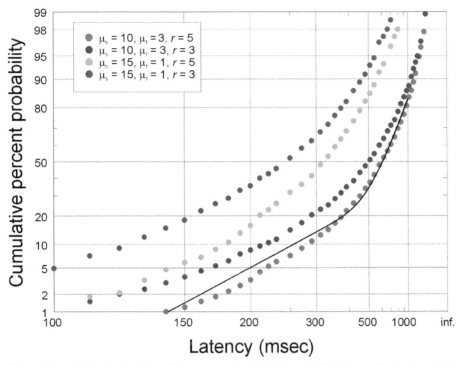

Figure App 1.6 Distributions from difference counting: simulations of 1000 trials per distribution, with the parameters shown. The black line shows a best-fit LATER distribution (with early component) to the distribution for ($\mu_s = 10$, ($\mu_f = 3$, $r = 5$)).

combinations of the parameters; within quite tight constraints one can generate curves that are similar to recinormals, and can produce satisfactory fits with $N = 1000$ if an early component is included. However, lacking any particular theoretical grounding there is not much reason to prefer it to the recinormal distribution.

App 1.4.2 Weibull

Another pragmatic function, introduced by engineers as a way of parameterising the tendency of equipment to fail at an early or a late stage; lacking a clear theoretical basis it has little to recommend it as far as reaction times are concerned apart from the small number of parameters. The formula is

$$C(t) = 1 - e^{-(t/\tau)^c}, \qquad \text{(App 1.13)}$$

where τ is a time-scale parameter and c a shape parameter. As can be seen in Figure

App 1.8, although for small values of c the long-latency end is too rounded and satisfactory fits cannot be obtained, with larger values fairly good approximations to LATER with early components are generated, statistically acceptable for $N = 1000$.

App 1.5 Other Theoretical Distributions

App 1.5.1 Poisson Distribution

The simplest of all is the *Poisson distribution*, in which there are k successive trials per unit time with a probability p of success in any particular trial: thus, the average frequency of successes is $pk = \mu$ Hz. The occurrence of just one such event then sufficient to trigger a response, and the average latency will be $1/\mu$, with exponential form (another name for it is *exponential distribution*) Figure App 1.9 shows three such distributions for

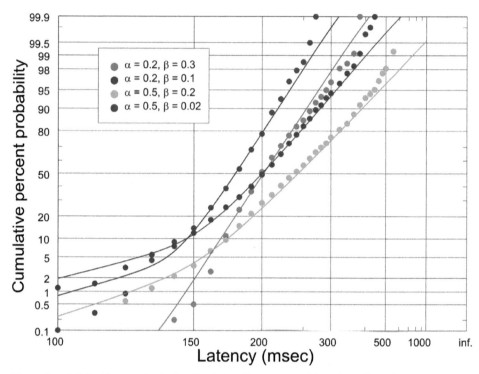

Figure App 1.7 The Normex distribution. Simulations for $\tau = 180$ and the values of α and β shown, with 1000 trials per run; the lines are best-fit LATER distributions, with early components.

different values of μ. Although, as noted earlier, the short-latency portion could serve as a generator of early saccades in conjunction with a LATER unit for the main distribution, the shapes of the distributions at the long-latency ends are quite unlike what is observed in real reaction time data.

App 1.5.2 Audley Distribution

The Audley distribution (Audley 1960) is given by

$$C(t) = 1 - \left(1 + \frac{t}{\tau}\right)e^{-t/\tau}, \qquad \text{(App 1.14)}$$

where the time-scaling parameter $\tau = 1/\alpha$. The resultant distributions are incompatible with LATER, even with an early component, because of the steep rise at the long-latency end (Figure App 1.10(a)).

App 1.5.3 Kintsch Distribution

Kintsch (Kintsch 1963) models latency as a random walk with random durations for each step, exponentially distributed. The resultant cumulative function is

$$C(t) = 1 - \frac{1}{(1-b)}\left(e^{\frac{-bt}{\tau}} - be^{\frac{-t}{\tau}}\right),$$

$$\text{(App 1.15)}$$

where τ is a time-scaling parameter, and b is a shape parameter. It is difficult to find values for these parameters that generate plausible distributions: Figure App 1.10(b) shows an attempt to do so, with and without and added transport delay; even with an early component it seems to be impossible to generate distributions that are compatible with LATER, mostly because of the very steep ascent at the long-latency end.

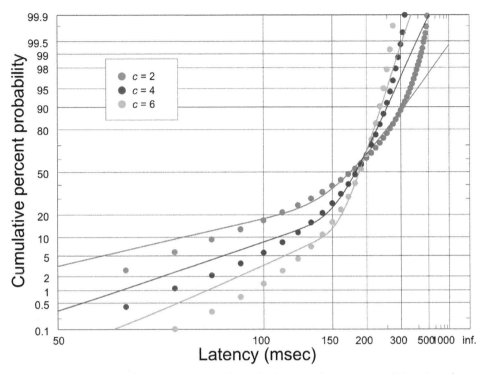

Figure App 1.8 The Weibull distribution. 1000 trials per distribution, with $\tau = 200$ ms and the values of c as shown: the lines showing best-fit LATER functions including early components.

App 1.5.4 Random Walk

This has often been proposed in one form or another (Stone 1960, Laming 1968, Watson 1979, Pacut 1980), and has been particularly carefully discussed by (Laming 1973) and promoted more recently particularly by Ratcliff (Ratcliff 1978, Ratcliff, van Zandt et al. 1999). The underlying model is of a signal rising towards a threshold θ at a rate that fluctuates from moment to moment with mean μ and variance σ^2. It has strong theoretical reasons to commend it, since it can be taken to embody a sequential likelihood test, the most efficient way of implementing a detection task (Wald and Wolfowitz 1948); this does not mean that it is equally appropriate for making the decision itself. There are two independent parameters, (μ/θ) and (σ/θ) (or, more usefully, (θ/μ) which is a characteristic time, and (μ/σ) which is a pure number). For the purpose of comparison with the recinormal distribution, (θ/μ) can be disregarded, since alterations in its value only cause a change in time-scale, that can be matched by corresponding changes in μ.

Figure App 1.11 shows reciprobit plots of a number of simulations of a random walk process, for $\mu = 5$ Hz and different values of σ. For a large number of trials, the resultant simulations produce distinctly curved lines, and do not fit the recinormal distribution unless (μ/σ) is very large. Empirical simulation suggests that the number of trials required to provide a significance level of $p = 0.05$ is given approximately by $N = 2800 \, (\mu/\sigma)^2$.

In other words, with small data sets the merits of the two distributions are indistinguishable; but with data sets of the order of a thousand the curvature of the random-walk plots becomes obvious.

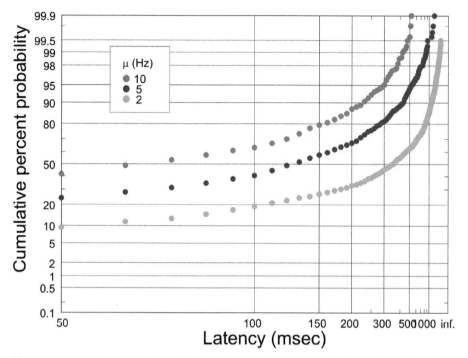

Figure App 1.9 Poisson distribution plotted as reciprobits for the values of μ shown: Monte Carlo simulation, 1000 trials per distribution.

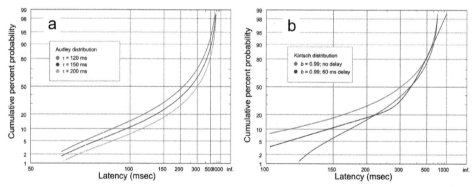

Figure App 1.10 (a) Audley distributions with β = 0 and the values of τ shown; (b) Kintsch distributions with τ = 200 ms, b = 0.99, and also with a transport delay of 60 ms; the black line shows the best-fit LATER fit, with an early component, to the latter.

App 1.5.5 Micko

Proposed by Micko (1969) on rather abstract theoretical grounds, relating to psychological scaling in general rather than modelling stochastic events, this distribution has a particularly simple cumulative form:

$$C(t) = \frac{1}{1 + (\tau/t)^c}, \tag{App 1.16}$$

where τ is the median latency, and c is a dimensionless factor that determines the shape. Despite the small number of parameters, the resultant curves (Figure App 1.12)

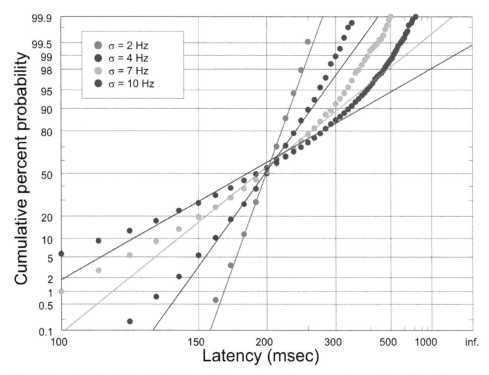

Figure App 1.11 Simulations (4000 trials each) of a random walk process with μ = 5 Hz and four different values of σ as shown; the lines show corresponding best-fit recinormal functions.

can be made to look very like a recinormal distribution with an early sub-population, except that with smaller values of c, at longer latencies the curves turn up too quickly.

App 1.5.6 Flat

A flat distribution, with a constant probability of occurrence between limits T and $T + W$ would result from a simple sampling model driven by a clock of constant interval W, and with transport delay T (see for example Carpenter 1988). However. it generates a reciprobit plot (Figure App 1.13(a)) with a shape quite unlike what is ever observed.

App 1.5.7 Gaussian

A Gaussian distribution, as might for instance result from a rise at constant rate to a threshold that varies in a Gaussian

manner, produces reciprobit plots that are too curved (Figure 1.13(b)) unless the variance is very small. It is possible to combine the idea of Gaussian variation of the threshold with a rise profile that is not linear, but chosen to get the right distribution (see, for example, Grice, Nullmeyer et al. 1977); if the function chosen is sufficiently close to a reciprocal, then such a model will behave indistinguishably from LATER. However, since in the general case such a model has at least five parameters, it is not so surprising that it can be made to fit real data very well, particularly considering that it includes the recinormal function in its repertoire.

App 1.5.8 Logistic

Finally, the logistic function has much to recommend it in the context of the

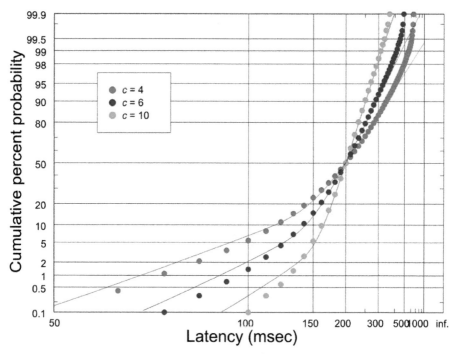

Figure App 1.12 The Micko distribution, with τ = 200 ms and c = 4, 6, and 10. The lines are best-fit LATER distributions, with early components.

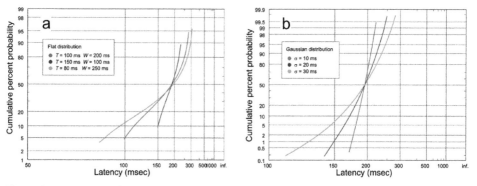

Figure App 1.13 (a) Flat distributions, with the values of T and W shown. (b) Gaussian distributions, with means of 200 ms and the values of the standard deviations as shown.

theory of the detection of signals; its cumulative is

$$C(x) = 1/\left(1 + e^{\frac{\mu - x}{\sigma}}\right). \qquad \text{(App 1.17)}$$

Over quite a wide range is remarkably similar in shape to a Gaussian. Consequently a reciprobit plot of a 'recilogistic' function – the logistic of reciprocal latency – gives a good straight line in the middle, but has curves in the tails (Figure App 1.14(b)), though still giving acceptable fits to LATER with $N = 1000$. Since it has some attractive mathematical properties – it has to be regarded as a perfectly viable alternative to LATER.

The overall conclusion must be that if a wide range of data is taken, most of the well-known theories are inadequate unless allowed several parameters, a conclusion previously arrived at by Vickers (1980) on a much more restricted range of data. On the other hand, the recinormal distribution, which Vickers could not have known of, appears to out-perform them all.

App 1.6 Combinations of Elements

App 1.6.1 Fixed Delay in Series

An unexpected feature of the recinormal distribution is how little it is affected by the addition of a moderate constant delay. Figure App 1.15(a) shows the effect of adding various fixed delays δ to a distribution having median latency of 150 ms. In the middle, various combinations of δ and T_M are used, such that the overall median latency is 200 ms. As can be seen, apparent linearity is preserved provided δ is not too large, and satisfactory fits are obtained so long as δ/μ is less than about 0.06, even though the function then looks noticeably curved. The effect of the delay δ is of course to increase the median latency by δ, and the apparent value of k by a factor of approximately $(1 + \delta\mu)$.

This robustness with respect to transport delay is an important result from the point of view of modelling the underlying latency mechanism, for it means that we

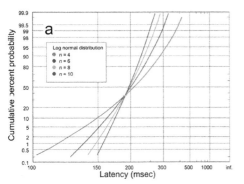
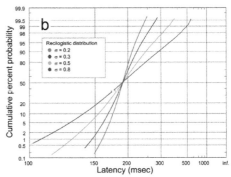

Figure App 1.14 (a) Log normal distributions, with the values of n shown, and $\tau = 200$ ms. (b) Recilogistic distributions (logistic functions of reciprocal reaction time) with values of σ as shown.

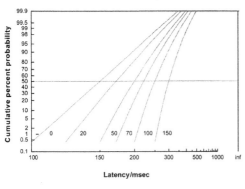
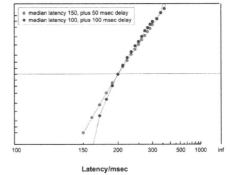

Figure App 1.15 Delay in series with a recinormal process. (a) Distributions resulting from adding delays δ of 0, 20, 50, 70, 100, or 150 ms in series with a recinormal process with $(\mu, \sigma) = (6.67, 1.26)$. In simulations with 2000 trials, only the cases of $\delta = 100$ and 150 fail the KS test. (b) Simulations with $N = 1000$ of a recinormal process with a median latency of 150 ms together with a delay of 50 ms, and with median latency of 100 ms and delay 100.

need not be much concerned with what can be an embarrassment for some theories, namely, the obvious fact that one (series) component of reaction time must inevitably be the peripheral delay that arises through nerve conduction, synaptic delays, receptor activation and muscle operation, but which together generate values for δ/μ that are well within the 0.06 limit.

App 1.6.2 Two Recinormal Processes in Series

Similarly, two recinormals in series produce reciprobit plots that are for all practical purposes indistinguishable from a single recinormal having the same overall median latency and slope (Figure App 1.16), and provide satisfactory fits provided that the values of μ for neither component exceeds 10 or so. In the limit, if the slope of one of them is infinite, we have the case of fixed delay previously

considered, for which the limitations have already been noted. The consequence is that in experiments with realistic numbers of trials, it is not possible to distinguish statistically between the operation of a single recinormal process and that of two (or more) in series.

App 1.6.3 Prior Dichotomy

Putting two stochastic processes, each with a unimodal latency distribution, in parallel does not generate a bimodal distribution overall, because of pre-emption. Yet latency distributions with dual or even multiple peaks are often found, at least for saccadic latencies (Fischer and Boch 1983, Fischer and Ramsperger 1984). To explain them, one needs to precede the parallel elements with a stochastic dichotomiser, a device that randomly enables just one of the elements on each trial. Provided the difference in the medians of the components is sufficiently large in relation to their

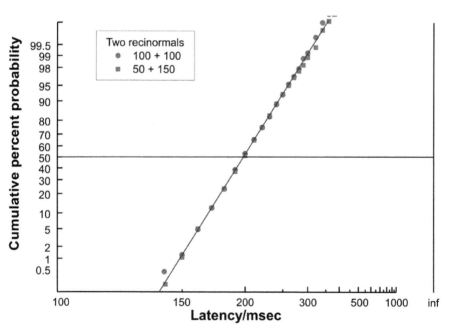

Figure App 1.16 Two recinormals in series. Simulations with ($N = 1000$) for two identical recinormals in series, each with median latency = 100 ms (red), and for one with 50 ms and one with 150 (blue), compared with the expectation for a single recinormal with 200 ms (blue line).

widths, the result will be a bimodal histogram. On a reciprobit plot, the curve moves from the asymptote that represents the faster process to the one that represents the slower (Chapter 2, Figure 2.7), and if the faster process is chosen on $P\%$ of trials, then provided the two medians are sufficiently far apart the curve will tend to flatten along the $P\%$ line in the middle. Note incidentally that in these raw histograms, generated from processes that cannot possibly give more than two peaks, how easy it is when looking at raw rather than cumulative histograms to imagine extra peaks where none in truth exists, simply as the result of chance statistical fluctuation.

This clear-cut difference between recinormals in parallel with or without prior dichotomy helps to elucidate the mechanisms giving rise to the deviation from a single recinormal often seen at the fast end of the distribution. In the case of saccades, express saccades form a sub-population that is frequently bimodal, generating reciprobit plots characteristic of parallel processes with prior dichotomy (Chapter 2, Figure 2.7). Other reaction times do not generally show bimodality, but often give reciprobit plots with a sub-population of early responses, corresponding to a reciprobit process in parallel with the main distribution, with $k = 0$. The clearest evidence that express responses and early responses are separate entities can be found in the responses that some subjects make in saccadic gap tasks, where the distribution appears to consist of both express and early responses, each sub-population being clearly identifiable in reciprobit plots (Chapter 2, Figure 2.8). The early responses are in some ways similar to what some authors call 'anticipatory' responses(Kalesnykas and Hallett 1987), but are distinguished from them by the fact that they are not simply random guesses; though a

proportion of them are often incorrect, and a higher proportion than for the main distribution, this proportion is typically much smaller than 50% (Carpenter 2001) .

App 1.7 Scales for Encoding Probability

Before going further, we need to think a little about how we actually assign numerical values to subjective probabilities in particular. How can we attach numbers to what we feel?

It was this question that drove the development of psychophysics, particularly in nineteenth-century Germany (Wundt 1862, Helmholtz 1867, Mach 1886, Wundt 1887). It was clear that when a subject was asked to assign a number to the magnitude of their perceptions – in effect, how they felt about different stimuli – in general these numbers were not simply proportional to the underlying physical measures.

An example is using the expansion of fluids to provide a scale of temperature. In some situations, a physical attribute like this does indeed provide a reliable scale that correlates with perception, but in other cases it does not. In general, a graded quantitative phenomenon can be represented on any of an infinite number of possible scales. Physical scales are necessarily arbitrary, provided two basic criteria are met. Formally, if the phenomenon at some moment has a value S_A on a physical scale A and generates a sensation judged by the subject to be S_B on scale B, we can express the relation between the two scales as a mapping function $S_B = f(S_A)$. The function f can be quite arbitrary, though if the scale is to be useful, it must be *monotonic*: the slope of the function must have the same sign throughout its range (Figure App 1.17). If we order a set of values by their size in one scale, the order should be the same in the other scale. (This is in fact disobeyed by several

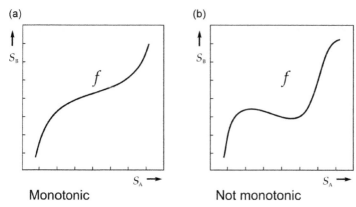

(a) Monotonic

(b) Not monotonic

Figure App 1.17 (a) A monotonic relation between two probability scales; (b) a non-monotonic relation.

sensory systems, notably in the phenomenon of paradoxical cold (Carpenter and Reddi 2012)). Finally, if a subjective scale is to be used to compare different perceptual magnitudes, there must be an agreed procedure for anchoring it to some kind of objective standard. In the case of temperature, for instance, the freezing and boiling points of water provide such a universal, objective reference. Assuming observers are capable of comparing one stimulus with another, statements like 'this is hotter than boiling water' will be correctly understood.

App 1.7.1 Non-linear Scales

The kind of statement that will not be universally understood, and will therefore be meaningless, is 'this is half as hot as boiling water', or even 'this is exactly halfway between boiling water and ice'. Even if we happen to have a physical scale – based, perhaps, on the idea that degree of expansion is a measure of temperature – it by no means follows that a cup of tea at 60° will feel twice as hot as one at 30°.

A well-studied example of a subjective scale is the highly non-linear relationship between luminance (in effect, a physical measure proportional to the rate at which photons enter the eye from a luminous surface) and the subjective sense of how bright the surface appears to be. Many kinds of psychophysical experiments, including directly asking people to rate brightness on a numerical scale or asking them to adjust the brightness of a surface until it seems twice as bright as some other surface, have demonstrated that – within limits – the relationship between perceived brightness and luminance is approximately logarithmic: $S = k \log(I)$, where I is the luminance of the source and S is a measure of the perceived brightness. This relationship is also suggested by measuring *increment thresholds*. Starting with some fixed background luminance, I, we suddenly add to it ΔI. We then ask the subject to reduce ΔI until it can only just be perceived. If we do this at different background luminances, we find that over a wide range, ΔI is proportional to the luminance I, so that $\Delta I / I$ is constant. This relationship (the Weber–Fechner law (Fechner 1860)) can easily be explained if we make the assumption that on the internal, subjective, scale, the threshold for perceiving a change is fixed. We can work out how this threshold, ΔS, relates to the observed increment threshold ΔI by differentiating our equation embodying the scaling relationship, yielding $dS/dI = k/I$. By rearranging, we then get $dI/I = dS/k$. From this it follows

(a)

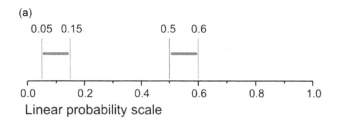

(b)

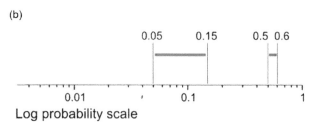

Figure App 1.18 The subjective effect of a given change in probability (in this case, from 0.05 to 0.15 (a), or alternatively from 0.5 to 0.6) may be very different if a log scale is used (b).

that provided the increments are not too big, $\Delta I/I$ will be constant.

Can we approach the problem of subjective probability scales in a similar way? A scale for probability that is linear with respect to frequency clearly has many advantages. It means that we can immediately calculate the probabilities of compound hypotheses, as, for example, being dealt a bridge hand that is entirely of one suit. On the other hand, rather as in the case of the perception of brightness, it does not really correspond to how we feel about probabilities. A change of probability from 0.5 to 0.6 does not seem as great as a change from say 0.05 to 0.15; and a change from 0 to 0.1 seems almost infinitely big, since complete impossibility feels qualitatively different from even a remote possibility, Figure App 1.18. As with brightness, could some kind of log scale be a better representation of how it feels? Going from $p = 0.5$ to 0.6 represents a ratio of 1.2, or 0.079 on a $\log_{10}$) scale, whereas going from 0.05 to 0.15 is a ratio of three and thus 0.48 on a log scale – about six times larger; and the jump from 0 to 0.1 is, in logarithmic terms, infinite.

App 1.7.2 Encoding Firmness of Belief

Beautiful though Bayes' Law is, human decisions are at best only partially Bayesian. As we saw in Section 3.4.1, we tend not to take sufficient account of prior probabilities. But there are at least two other ways in which Bayes' cannot provide a complete account of how we make decisions. The first is that it does not take into account the different *values* of different hypotheses, when they turn out to be true. In the case of the urns, for instance, if we were told that the prize for correctly guessing the first urn was ten times bigger than the prize for correctly guessing the second, our behaviour ought (if we are rational) to be guided not so much by what we believe to be true, but what will lead to the biggest reward. This extremely important topic is considered at greater length in Chapter 6, Section 6.3. But even leaving reward aside, there is another aspect that certainly modifies the way we actually make decisions, namely, *firmness* of belief, a measure of how easily prior probabilities are modified by fresh evidence.

In the classical Bayes formula, E is a definite event, known for certainty. How should the formula be modified if it is only known *probabilistically*? All sensory signals are transmitted via noisy channels. The observation of E is itself a hypothesis for which afferent signals provide evidence. For a neuron, there is no distinction between hypotheses and events. Unfortunately, analysis of even the simplest cases doesn't lead to simple answers: it is not simply that support ought to be multiplied by the firmness of belief in the evidence (or at least its probability). A single parameter is inadequate to describe one's feelings about a future event. Suppose we have a bag known to contain only black beans and white beans, and we take out two of them: one is black, one white. So, our first estimate will be that p(white) = 0.5. and p(black) also= 0.5. But if we sample a hundred, and 50 are black and 50 white, our belief that p(white) = 0.5 and p(black) = 0.5 is evidently much stronger. This is not a problem for the brain, which tends to work by activity in parallel. Thus, we can have simultaneous activity in a neuron whose activity represents belief in a hypothesis and in its contrary, with no necessary relationship between the two. After the second sample, both will be more active than before.

Now a benefit of odds (App 1.7.4), expressed as a pair of numbers such as (2:3) rather than literally as a fraction (2/3), is that they build up with experience as 'favourable' and 'unfavourable' cases, so that their ratio becomes more robust as more experience is gathered. A single observation will have a large effect on (1:1) because it is easily modified; less so on (1000:1000). It also means that incoming information may alter the robustness of these pairs without affecting the odds themselves, as when (1/1), after many observations, may become (1000/1000). Finally, this approach also helps solve the problem of indifference: if nothing is known, we get (0/0), which is undefined.

One mechanism could be to run races between H and ~H. Slower means more variable, so that a vaguer belief is more easily swayed by other circumstances. In isolation, there would be no difference between a firm belief in p = 0.5 and a vague one; in both cases, one would expect to act as if H were true on half the occasions.

But how should our feeling that a probability is more vague or less vague affect our behaviour? Imagine two urns, A and B, each with a different mixture of 100 black and red balls. With replacement, I choose two from A: one is red, the other black; then I choose four balls from B: two are red and two are black. Now I am told to select either A or B and choose a ball from it: if it is red, I win a prize. Which urn should I choose? Bayes says they are equally good, since the priors and likelihoods are identical. But since we know for certain that A has at least one red ball, and B at least two, one could argue that one should choose B. On the other hand, this is equally true if the prize is for drawing black rather than red – again, one should choose B! So, in response to vagueness, other things being equal, we should choose whatever hypothesis is least vague, because this maximises expected utility. If a coin comes heads 10 times in 10 tosses, we still believe it unbiased; if a treatment cures 10/10 patients, we believe it works, even though its prior probability might be 0.5 (Lindley 1956, Dempster 1968). The difference lies in the form of the prior distribution in each case: if it is bimodal, for example, a penny we know either to be biased 0.4 or 0.6 (Lindley 1956).

Is there any reason to include probability vagueness as intrinsic part of probability theory? Ordinary measurements are equally subject to hierarchies of uncertainties – *all* numbers have an implied vagueness about them. Consider 'This plank is 1 m long' and 'This plank is 1.2 m long' and 'This plank is 1.2305 m long', implying their different degrees of precision.

So, what we need is a measure of *certainty*, in other words of the probability that the current probability might change through receipt of further information.

App 1.7.3 Simple Log Scale

This suggests that we could use, say, $U(A) = 1/p(A)$ to represent subjective probability, or rather, subjective *uncertainty*, for the larger U is, the more uncertain we are that the event in question will occur. It doesn't much matter what base we use for our logarithm, as all this does is apply an arbitrary scaling factor. There is something to be said for using a base of 2 when we consider its close relation to measures of information (bits).

Apart from corresponding to how we feel, there is another advantage of a log scale. To calculate the probability of a composite event, like throwing two sixes, or picking two winners in a race, we use multiplication: if we toss two coins, the probability of two heads is ¼, of three is 1/8. But on a log scale this corresponds to simple addition. The probability of throwing heads in a single toss is 0.5, so $U = 1$; the probability of throwing two heads in two tosses is 0.25, so U is 2; and of throwing N heads in N tosses is simply N. In a similar vein, we can calculate that the uncertainty before throwing a six with two dice is 5.17, or about the same as for 5 coin tosses; before drawing an ace from a pack of cards $U = 3.7$; and just before the main draw of the UK National Lottery U is about 25 – in other words, the probability of your chosen set of numbers being drawn is about the same as of throwing 25 heads in succession. This provides a handy, intuitive feel for different degrees of probability: hat the scale has a basic unit of one coin toss, a degree of

uncertainty with which we are tolerably familiar. $U(A)$ is the same as (Good 1955, Good 1971) Good's $I(A)$ and also (Jeffreys 1931) Jeffreys' improbability, $imp(A) = 1/p(A)$ (see App 1.1.2).

One aspect of this simple log scale is not quite right: it is that U must apply to a collection, not to individual potential events. It only works in cases where we don't know which of a number of equal possibilities will occur. In a sense, it is a measure not so much of what we feel before the event, but the change in our feeling – something like the degree of surprise – when the event occurs. If there are two possible events A and B, of probability $p(A)$ and $p(B) = (1 - p)$, and p is quite large, then we are going to be less surprised when A happens than when B happens. Since A will happen more often, the expected degree of surprise ought to be something like $-p \log(p + (1 - p) \log(1 - p))$ – the sum of the surprises for each possible outcome, weighted by the probabilities of their actually occurring. In general, with a set of N different possible events of different probabilities, the prior uncertainty, or expected surprise, will be $\Sigma(p_i \log(p_i))$. The concept of surprise is an interesting one, and deeply related to experimental design (Section 6.2.1 in Chapter 6).

But there is something fundamentally wrong with it. Unlike luminance, probability is strictly bounded at both ends, 1 and 0. Furthermore, since any information gained about p is also gained about $(1 - p)$, the function must be symmetrical in p and $(1 - p)$: for any proposition A, $p(A)$ is necessarily equal to $(1 - p(\sim A))$. Intuitively, a change from $p = 0$ to 0.01 does indeed seem much bigger than, say, from 0.5 to 0.51, but so for that matter does a change from 0.99 to 1.00, which gives the least change in log p. Similarly, $p = 1$ seems qualitatively different from $p = 0.9999$. So, the subjective probability scale cannot in fact be simply be – log(*p*). Can we find an alternative?

App 1.7.4 Odds

One measure of probability that has the desired kind of symmetry is probably more familiar to the general public than *p* itself. When bookmakers express a horse's probability of winning, they do it in terms of the *odds*, a pair of numbers proportional to (1 – *p*) and *p*. In other words, an event that is judged to have a probability of 0.25 would be described as having odds of 3 to 1 (which can be written 3:1); high odds mean high improbability. (Conventionally, odds of 1:1 are called evens; and if *p* > 0.5, the odds are inverted: *p* = 0.75 is '3 to 1 against', or 1:3). Odds represent a proportion, so that odds of 4:2 are exactly the same as 2:1. They might in fact just well be written as a fraction, so that 2:1 becomes 1/2 (but see App 1.7.2) More formally, we can write that the odds in favour of some hypothesis H are given by *p*(H)/*p*(~H). A disadvantage of odds, as opposed to *p* or *U*, is that it does not lend itself easily to dealing with composite probabilities. Thus the odds of both A and B occurring, *p*(A . B), is given by an ugly expression: (*p*(A)/(1 – *p*(A))(*p*(B)/1 – *p*(B))/(1 + (*p*(A)/(1 – *p*(A)) + ((*p*(B)/(1 – *p*(B)).

App 1.7.5 Log Odds

Odds are desirably symmetrical, but don't embody the logarithmic feeling noted earlier. The final step is then to use the logarithm of the odds. This has been proposed independently, and for different reasons, by various authors, with correspondingly varied terminology (see App 1.1.2). The single most useful is Peirce's *belief* : bel(A) = log(*p*(A)/(1 – *p*(A)) = *U* (~A) – *U*(A). This scale goes from –∞ (impossible) to ∞ (inevitable): a coin toss, evens, being represented by zero. As we shall see, it has many admirable properties

that make it a good candidate for use by neurons in the brain, but it has the severe drawback that – like odds – it doesn't immediately provide a calculus for working out the probability of combined events. For instance, with two coin tosses the prior belief for two heads is log(0.25/0.75) or log(1/3) (about –1.099); but about 0.693 for a single toss. *U* is much simpler in this respect.

App 1.7.6 Information and Probability

Classical information theory (Good 1971) only deals with true hypotheses. The information received on discovering A is true is –log(*p*(A)) = *I*(A); none is received on discovering B is false unless there are only two alternatives, since it is equivalent to finding that ~B is true. For example, suppose in urn A half the balls are red and the rest black; in B, half are red and the rest various colours. If I draw a red ball from A, I also know it's not black; if from B, I know it's not blue, not green, not pink, and so on as well. Is the information gained the same?

$$\log \frac{p(\mathrm{H|E})}{p(\mathrm{H})} = \log \frac{p(\mathrm{E|H})}{p(\mathrm{E})}$$
$$= \log \frac{p(\mathrm{E.H})}{p(\mathrm{E})p(\mathrm{H})} = I(\mathrm{E : H})$$
$$= I(\mathrm{H : E})$$

Like probability, and information, 'noise' is also a subjective matter, like deciding whether a plant in your garden is a 'weed'. So, information may not necessarily improve our estimates of probability. Think of Ali Baba and the 40 thieves: a thief marks a victim's door with chalk: the victim responds by marking *all* the doors. We really want a function of *p* that asymptotes upwards at the edges, for instance, 1/(*p*(1 – *p*)). In fact, we need to distinguish *Fisher* information (which is the same as Edwards (2000) *expected* information), *Shannon* information, which is a measure of the maximum amount of information a channel can convey (Shannon and Weaver 1949), and observed information (Edwards 1992). Fisher information is closely related to entropy in the thermodynamic sense (Fisher 1935), though he realised that there were 'profound differences'.

App 1.7.7 Surprise

Different measures of surprise have been proposed, and they are summarised in App 1.1.2. The simplest is Good's: sex(X) = $\mathscr{E}(p)/p$, the ratio of the expected – long-term average – probability to the actual probability But shouldn't this depend on a preconception as to what series would in fact be surprising? In other words, surprise is just as much a subjective and personal matter as noise, information, and probability itself. On this basis, HTHT is just as surprising as HHHH – as indeed it is, if that was what was predicted in advance.

'Surprise' depends on perceived patterns and meanings: like throwing a six when a six was predicted, for which sex = 13/3 – same as throwing a double (as it should be), Figure App 1.19.

In binary cases like these (i.e., either as predicted – probability = p – or not), sex = ($2p$ – 2 + 1/p).

For example, '*I'm going to throw three heads*' – then they do exactly that: so sex = 25/4.

So, 6 = remarkable; 4 = strange; 1 = exactly as expected. However, this breaks down if p = 1/2 (e.g., predicting a head, does it): gives sex = 1. Or indeed if we specify one of a number of equiprobable things in advance, like a roulette score, sex = 1!

App 1.7.8 Single Hypotheses

Neurons care nothing for truth: fuzziness.

$$\frac{P'(H)}{P'(\overline{H})} = \frac{P(S|H)}{P(S|\overline{H})} \cdot \frac{P(H)}{P(\overline{H})}.$$

There are several proposed ways in which neuronal spikes are signalling occurrence of new information (Deneve 2008), as illustrated in Figure App 1.20.

App 1.8 Modelling Choice

Once we have some conception of how individual neurons, or pairs of neurons, code for the probability of hypotheses, we can try to explain how overall decisions are arrived at. In general, we expect some kind of race between units, such that better-supported hypotheses tend to be chosen, and that this is modulated by a random process that is most evident when the probabilities of the competing hypotheses are most similar.

App 1.8.1 Pre-emption

With two race-to-threshold elements, if one is substantially faster than the other it will 'win' nearly every time and pre-empt the contribution of the slower one,

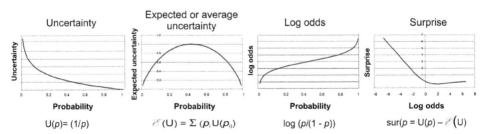

Figure App 1.19 Surprise, and related measures, as a function of probability or log odds.

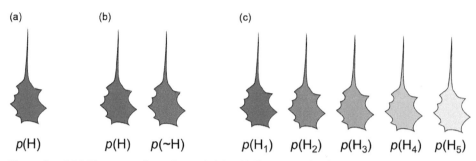

Figure App 1.20 Three ways of encoding probability. (a) The activity of each neuron has a simple relationship to the probability it represents, $p(H)$. (b) Probability coded by a pair of neurons, one representing $p(H)$ and the other $p(\sim H)$. (c) A population of neurons coding for relative probabilities $p(H_1)$, $p(H_2)$, $p(H_3)$, etc.; in a race-to-threshold, the best supported will still win.

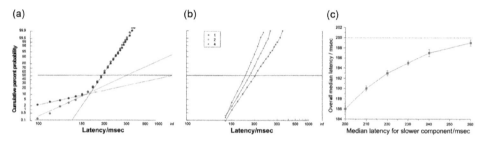

Figure App 1.21 Pre-emption. (a) Simulations ($N = 2000$) of (left) a recinormal with $(\mu, \sigma) = (5.00, 0.71)$ (black line) in parallel with a recinormal with $(\mu, \sigma) = (3.40, 2.24)$ (red) and with an early component with $k = 0$ (blue). (b) 1, 2, or 4 identical recinormals $(\mu, \sigma) = (5.00, 0.71)$ in parallel. (c) Reduction in median latency caused by having a recinormal with $(\mu, \sigma) = (5.00, 0.71)$ in parallel with another, slower recinormal with the same value of k but different medians, as shown.

which will not have a chance to influence more than slightly the overall distribution of the latency. As a result, the overall distribution is not, as might be thought, bimodal; indeed, if the component elements are recinormals, it turns out that the overall distribution is also very similar to that of a single recinormal. This is a standard way of modelling express saccades (see Chapter 2, Section 2.2.2). Figure App 1.21 shows some examples, using simulations with 2000 trials in each run; in each case, there is one element with $(\mu, \sigma) = (5.00, 0.71)$, and one or more with different parameters operating in parallel. The case with $k = 0$ is interesting as it provides a close simulation of the small sub-population of early responses often observed in experimental data. It also shows what happens when two or more recinormals with identical parameters are arranged in parallel: the result is to reduce μ and increase k, the lines remaining essentially straight, and simulations are within the $p = 0.05$ for KS, with $N = 1000$ though not for 2000. The effect of a second recinormal with a different μ falls off as the difference increases, and if one is more than 25% greater than the other its effect is negligible.

App 1.8.2 Races between Cooperative Pairs of LATER Units

There are two situations where LATER units may race in parallel: if they are responsible for different responses, then they are antagonistic; otherwise, they are cooperative. In the first case, we will get

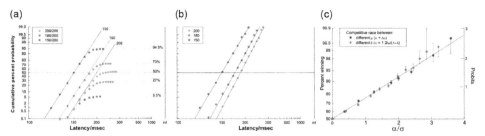

Figure App 1.22 Cooperative elements in parallel. (a) Simulations (*N* = 2047) of cooperative recinormal processes, one having (μ, σ) = (5.00, 0.71), and the other having *k* = 7 and median latencies of 150, 180, or 200 ms. The lines show the expected distributions for the individual processes on their own, the points show incomplete reciprobit plots (percentages of the total number of trials). (b) Complete reciprobit plots of the same data (percentages of the number of favourable trials only). (c) Percentage of 2000 trials in which a recinormal with smaller μ wins against another of identical *k*, plotted on a probability scale as a function of α/σ, where α = Δμ, the difference between the two values of μ (red), or against one of identical μ and *k* that is delayed by δ (blue); in this case, α = 1.2δ μ/(μ + δ). The solid line is for probability in probits = Δμ/σ√2.

different responses, depending on which unit won; in the second case, the response will always be the same, but in general the latency will be reduced (unless there is significant lateral inhibition: see Chapter 4, Section 4.4). There are many situations, as in a classical choice reaction time experiment, where the parallel elements generate different responses. In a competitive race of this kind, the latency behaviour of the individual elements determines not only the latency distribution of the system as a whole, but also the final choice. Under these conditions, a reciprobit plot of the latency of one of the responses, with the cumulative percentage expressed as a fraction of all trials, has a characteristic shape (Figure App 1.22). This shows the results of pitting a recinormal with μ = 5.00 against one with μ = 5.55 or μ = 6.66, all with the same value of *k* = 7. The lines show the expected distributions for each element on its own, and the points are plotted for each response with both elements competing together. It can be seen that, in general, each curve starts along the asymptote provided by its own recinormal line, and then turns over relatively abruptly to level off at a percentage representing the final

frequency of that response; this is true for the slower element as well as the faster.

A further, surprising, instance of the robustness of the reciprobit plot is that if the results are plotted taking the cumulations as percentages of only those trials where that response was made (so that each necessarily reaches 100%), the result is a very nearly straight line and generates KS values well within the *p* = 0.05 limit for *N* = 2000 (Figure App 1.22). A similar result is found if the two responses are simply pooled (this is simply the non-competitive case previously discussed). The percentage of trials on which the faster process wins depends on the parameters of the two distributions. In the situation discussed so far, on a probit scale there appears to be a linear relation to Δμ, the difference between the two values of μ; in fact, the frequency in probits is given by Δμ/σ. The same general relationship seems to hold for the case where the two processes are identical, but one is started at a time δ after the other: a handicap race (precedence task). Figure App 1.22(c) shows probability in probits (see the data in Chapter 4, Section 4.5.1) where β = 1.2 provides the best fit to the data.

App 1.8.3 Races between Antagonistic Pairs of LATER Units

A common situation is one of two competing LATER units, (μ_1, σ_1) and (μ_2, σ_2). What is the proportion of wins by the faster one as a function of the parameters? In simpler cases, this can be determined analytically, and we repeat here a simplified version of the analysis set out in (Noorani and Carpenter 2016).

If we have (μ_1, σ_1) racing against (μ_2, σ_2), plotting the promptness of one against the other over a number of trials will generate a bivariate distribution (Figure App 1.23(b)), with unit 1 winning when the corresponding point lies to the left of the line $(\lambda_1 = \lambda_2)$. We can scale the resultant ellipse to make it circular (Figure App 1.23(c)).

Now unit 1 wins when the point lies to the left of $(\sigma_1 y = \sigma_2 x)$. The distance of this line from the centre of the distribution is $\frac{\Delta\mu}{\sqrt{\sigma_1^2 + \sigma_2^2}}$, where $\Delta\mu = \mu_1 - \mu_2$

Therefore, the required probability

$$p = P\left(\frac{\Delta\mu}{\sqrt{\sigma_1^2 + \sigma_2^2}}\right).$$

For the special case of $\sigma_1 = \sigma_2$,

$$p = P\left(\frac{\Delta\mu}{\sigma\sqrt{2}}\right);$$ we can relate this to the reciprobit plot by drawing the asymptotic lines separately (Figure App 1.24): if we put $\xi = (\Delta\mu / \sigma)$, then the vertical distance between them is.

So, to find the horizontal asymptote, representing the required proportion of successes for unit 1 in the presence of unit 2, draw a vertical line from μ_2 to intersect the distribution for unit 1, and scale by a

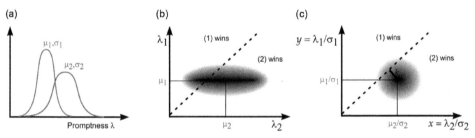

Figure App 1.23 (a) Two competing units with different values of μ and σ. (b) Together, they generate an elliptical bivariate distribution. (c) With suitable scaling, the distribution will be circular rather than elliptic. The dashed line represents the division between trials where μ_1 wins and where μ_2 wins.

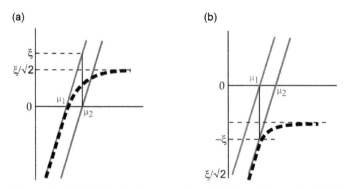

Figure App 1.24 (a) To find the proportion of trials in which μ_1 wins, find the point (μ_2, ξ): then the required proportion is $\xi/\sqrt{2}$. Similarly (b), to find the proportion of trials in which μ_2 wins, find the point (μ_2, ξ); $\xi/\sqrt{2}$ will again be the required proportion.

factor $1/\sqrt{2}$. Conversely, to find the horizontal asymptote for unit 2 in the presence of unit 1, draw a vertical line from μ_1 to intersect the distribution for unit 2, and scale by $1/\sqrt{2}$.

App 1.8.4 Bayesian Races

The problem may also be approached from a Bayesian perspective. Suppose we have two hypotheses H_1 and H_2, which need not be mutually exclusive, and some evidence E; let the probability of getting result E on hypothesis H be $p(E|H)$. Then the likelihood of H given E is $L(H|E), = kp (E|H)$ where k is an arbitrary constant (Fisher 1921), which then cancels out. So the likelihood ratio is then $L(H_1|E)/L(H_2| E)$; the log of this quantity has been called the *weight of the evidence* afforded by E $(W (H_1/H_2: E))$ in favour of H_1 as compared with H_2 (Good 1950, Good 1968, Good 1975):

$$W(H_1/H_2 : E) = \log L(H_1, H_2|E)$$
$$= \log p(E|H_1) - \log p(E|H_2),$$
$$\text{(App 1.18)}$$

with the advantage that the combined weight of two pieces of evidence is simply the sum of their individual weights.

App 1.8.5 Races between Many LATER Units

If we have a large set of possible hypotheses (for instance, the possible existence of several stimulus objects), we do not want to have to compare each with every other one in pairs. Rise-to-threshold provides a means of simultaneously comparing all hypotheses and selecting the most likely one, if each decision signal is taken as a measure of the belief B_j in an associated hypothesis H_j, where B_j is equal to $K + \log (L(H_j|T))$, and K is an arbitrary constant, so that the log-odds $\log(p(H_j)/(HL_j))$ of any pair of hypotheses is given by $(B_j - B_j)$. Figure App 1.25 represents a scheme of this kind; it has a set of hypotheses H_j and a selection E composed of a selection from m possible stimulus elements S_i, related by a matrix L_{ij} of the likelihoods $L(H_j|S_i)$. Thus the log-likelihood for H_j given E is $\Sigma_I (\log L_{ij})$, and the updated posterior belief is $B_j{}' = B_j + \Sigma_i(\log L_{ij})$

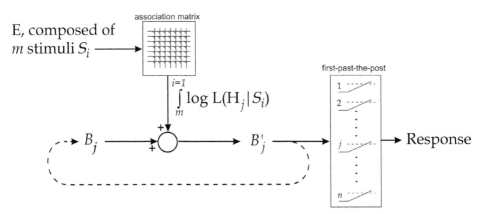

Figure App 1.25 Schematic representation of parallel multiple implementation of the rise-to-threshold model. A stimulus event E consists of the detection of a set of stimulus elements S_i, of which there are m. For each of a set of potential hypotheses H_j concerning the existence of particular targets, of which there are n, the sum of the weight of the evidence from E, is calculated from the learnt associations $p(S_i|H_j)$ between stimulus elements and hypotheses, and used to update the corresponding belief function B_j. This process continues until one of the B_j reaches a criterion level, at which point the appropriate response is initiated and all the B_j are reset.

If we are not interested in the odds for individual pairs of hypotheses, but only in the best overall hypothesis, then all we need do is run a race. B_j starts at some level representing the prior likelihood, and then, if updating occurs at constant intervals of time, E will rise at a rate proportional to the log of the likelihood ratio, until it reaches a criterion level which may be taken to represent a sufficient degree of belief to permit action. The dynamic properties of the model can be taken care of simply by arranging for feedback such that the B_j at time $t + 1$ is equal to B_j' at time t.

App 1.9 Learning

In Section 4.1 in Chapter 4, we saw that a change in prior probability in the middle of a run causes the reaction time on each side to alter in much the same way as a 'static' prior probability that is constant throughout the run. The time-course of this alteration appears to be roughly exponential, taking about 70 trials finally to settle down at the new equilibrium. It was pointed out there that the phenomenon is better considered as a process of forgetting, in that the contribution of old evidence gradually contributes less new, being discounted by what we called a Lethean factor λ, whose value is typically around 0.05. This is not, of course, how a strict Bayesian model should behave: all evidence, whether recent or not, should count equally. It is, however, relatively easy to model at the synaptic level, using a Hebbian-like mechanism.

An alternative formulation (Peirce 1878) just needs two opposed neurons coding for I(H) and I(~H), an event E increasing the firing of each in proportion to I(E|H) and I(E|~H) respectively. Synapses must therefore strengthen in proportion to Peircean probability of E with respect to H and ~H.

The distinction between 'probability' (for hypotheses) and 'chance' (for events)

unnecessary: both are talking about the same kind of neural activity: to a neuron, so an event *is* a hypothesis. It is also clear that probability and causation are the same kind of phenomenon. And so is perception itself: the reconstruction of the 'real' world is as much guesswork as the extrapolation into future possible worlds, and involves precisely similar neural processes. Though we tend to compare the uncertainty of the future with the certainty of the past, as every historian knows, we guess the past just as much as the future.

Probability is represented in two quite different ways: strengths of synapses represent conditional probabilities or likelihoods, while firing frequency represents degree of belief in a hypothesis. The patterns of activity of afferent synapses represent patterns of circumstantial support, while sub-threshold depolarisation represents prior probability represented. Then the Lethean factor λ (Chapter 4, Section 4.1) represents the speed with which synaptic strength can change.

App 1.9.1 Hebbian Synapses as Bayesian Computers

We have seen that in an uncertain world decisions are all about probability, and showed how sensory information is used as evidence and determines the strength of one's belief in hypotheses about the outside world, and how to quantify this process.

The final stage of this whole process is something called *confirmation*, which is at the heart of how neurons learn. So far, the various conditional probabilities $p(E|H)$ have been presented as if they were given, but of course they have to be learnt through experience, being themselves updated when the truth about whether the prediction was actually correct is finally revealed. This is exactly equivalent to the use of parametric feedback after the

(a)

UCS

CS

Naive

R
Salivation

(b)

UCS

CS

After conditioning)

R
Salivation

(c)

UCS

CS

A   X

B

R

(d)

A

B

X

Hebbian
synapse

Figure App 1.26 Highly simplified representation of Pavlovian conditioning. In the untrained animal there is an intrinsic, hard-wired link by which food (the unconditional stimulus, or UCS) causes salivation (a). After sufficient of food with a conditional stimulus (CS) such as a bell, the CS will trigger salivation even in the absence of food (b). The inescapable conclusion is that there are now two chains of neurons, from the CS and UCS, and that there must be at least one neuron (X) that is common to both (c). If this neuron shows Hebbian learning, its connection from the CS will be strengthened (d).

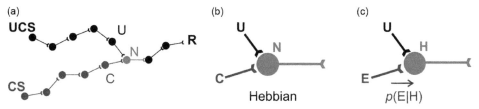

(a)

UCS

CS

U

N

C

R

(b)

U

N

C

Hebbian

(c)

U

H

E

$p(E|H)$

Figure App 1.27 (a) Chains of neurons connecting CS and UCs to the response R. (b) Neuron X has a Hebbian synapse ultimately driven by the CS. (c) If we identify U with a hypothesis H, and E with an observed event (the conditional stimulus CS), then the strength of the synapse ($p(E|U)$ represents likelihood and therefore embodies Bayesian learning:

event in motor control and is quite an enlightening way at looking at many kinds of learning.

Take the simplest of all – Pavlovian conditioning (Pavlov 1927), Figure App 1.26. After the conditioning has been learnt, the dog is in effect using the bell as evidence E for the hypothesis U that food is in the offing. And when it does finally appear, the value of $p(E|U)$, $p(bell|food)$ is increased. This updating or confirmation is what psychologists mean by reinforcement, but it is obviously an example of a Bayesian process as well.

Learning of this kind can be performed by Hebbian synapses (Hebb 1949), of which NMDA synapses are a well-known example. When they get stronger as a result of association between pre-synaptic and post-synaptic activity, this is equivalent to altering $p(E|H)$, so that next time the hypothesis is considered even more likely when the bell is heard, Figure App 1.27. Things that tend

to happen together in the outside world tend to get associated together in the brain: '*fire together, wire together*' We are building in our brain a model of probability relationships in the outside world, perpetually predicting what's coming next (Carpenter and Williams 1995, Brodersen, Penny et al. 2008), Figure App 1.28.

Can we work out what the rule for Hebbian strengthening (and weakening) must be if a synapse is to function as a Bayesian element? If it acts linearly, its strength S should be proportional to log $(p(U|C))$. Its history consists of the number of instances of U and C (n_{UCS}) occurring together, and the total number of instances of C on its own (n_C). Then $S = \log(n_{UC}/n_C)$.

So how must S change in response to C or UCS in order to generate this function? The answer is that after every occurrence of C the strength should decline by $\log(1 + 1/n_C)$, and if U occurs as well it

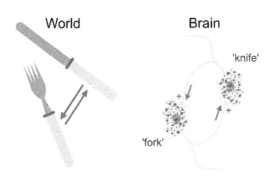

World   Brain   'knife'

'fork'

Figure App 1.28 Thanks to Hebbian synapses, the connections between neurons in the brain come to correspond to neural connections forming a model of the outside world.

should also increase by $\log (1 + 1/n_{UC})$. Since $\log (1 + x) = x - x^2/2 + x^3/3, \ldots$, to a first approximation the strength should change by $-1/n_C$ and $1/n_{UC}$, respectively. Unfortunately, this implies that the synapse needs to have a memory not only of its own strength, but also of its tally of UC and C events. This may sound unreasonable: what we want is an updating rule that uses only the current S and the fact of the event U&C or C. However, the overall strength of the synapse might be the result of *two* parameters representing independently the history of C and the history of UC. They could be the numbers of two different kinds of membrane channel, for example, NMDA versus AMPA: is it plausible that the total excitation could be a log function of the number of active channels? If $S = \log (n_{UCS}) - \log(n_C)$, then the rule could be extremely simple: after U&C, the number of each type of channel increases by one; after C alone, n_C increases by one. So, one might predict two sets of channels, one excitatory and increasing after conjunction, the other inhibitory and increasing after presynaptic activity only, though this is not in fact how AMPA and NMDA receptors behave. Physiologists will recognise that the formula for S is in effect the same as for the Nernst potential ($V = k(\log(C_1/C_2)$, where C_1 and C_2 are the numbers of each of the ions on each side of the membrane.

App 1.10 Information and Probability

App 1.10.1 Uncertainty as Lack of Information

Another conceivable scenario regarding the input of information regarding a hypothesis is that some information is provided about this hypothesis, but then a contradictory signal is given that cancels that previous message. Such conflicting input can be encoded as illustrated in Figure App 1.29.

App 1.10.2 Information in Extended Displays

In Section 4.6 in Chapter 4, we looked at various types of tasks in which the subject is required to make a judgement about whether in a field filled randomly with a mixture of two or more individual categories of discrete stimuli (for instance, red and green dots), there are more of one of the categories than the other. In the Type 1 version of this task, a proportion a of the total of N items are the same, while the remainder are random (for example, in an RDK experiment a dots may move consistently to the right, while the others execute a random walk). In a Type 2 version, there are a items of one kind (for example, moving to the right), and the remainder ($N - a$) are of the other kind, so that discrimination gets more difficult as a approaches ($N/2$). A simple

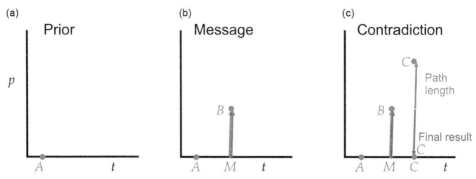

(a) Prior (b) Message (c) Contradiction

Figure App 1.29 (a) Initial probability for some hypothesis H. (b) A message is received telling us the value B of $p(H)$. (c) A second message is received, saying that the previous message was untrue. P reverts to its original (red), but the total path length is increased.

example of a Type 1 task was addressed in Reddi and Carpenter (2003). One needs to bear in mind that estimating the information content of such displays is not entirely straightforward and depends on certain assumptions, in particular on how local the estimation of direction of movement for any one of the detector units is. Here we assume it to be very local, as also have Weiss and Adelson (Weiss and Adelson 1998, Reddi, Asrress et al. 2003); the topic has been thoughtfully discussed by Barlow and Tripathy (Barlow and Tripathy 1997).

We start with the two opposed hypotheses, that at a particular moment the majority of dots are moving to the right (H_R) or to the left (H_L). Using Bayes, the observation E of one dot moving to the right will increase the log likelihood ratio for H_R versus H_L by log (C), where C is the likelihood ratio, $(p(E|H_R)/(pE|H_L)$.

In a Type 1 experiment, with N items, the probability of a particular item moving rightwards if H_R is true is $(aN + (N - aN)/2)/N$, or $(1 + a)/2$. Similarly, the

probability of an item moving leftwards if H_L is true is $(1 - a)/2$; so the likelihood ratio for any one item will be $C = (1 + a)/(1 - a)$: in many ways, C can be thought of as a kind of velocity contrast. The support for H_R against H_L for the entire display will be N log C, so in terms of LATER the median rate of rise of the decision signal be proportional to log (C). Then the median reaction time will be

$$T_0 + k/(N \log C),$$

where k is an arbitrary constant that is likely to vary from person to person, and T_0 is the constant delay encapsulating all those factors, such as conduction time, synaptic delay, and the time needed to activate muscle, that can be regarded as constant for any particular task. The larger a is, the shorter the reaction time will be.

In a Type 2 experiment, the difference is simply that the probability of observing a particular dot moving rightwards if H_R is true is a, but $(1 - a)$ if H_L is true. So, C is now given by $a/(1 - a)$.

Appendix 2 Clinical

That along with excitation of discharges of nervous arrangements in the cerebrum, mental states occur, I, of course, admit; but how this is I do not enquire; indeed, so far as clinical medicine is concerned, I do not care.

J. Hughlings Jackson, Selected Writings (1932)

Clinical neurology is currently a number-free zone (Antoniades and Carpenter 2012, Carpenter 2012). Compared with, say, haematology or cardiology we lack quantitative measures of impairment of response to treatment. One of the attractions of saccadometry – the measurement of saccadic latency distributions – is the wealth of very detailed quantitative information that it can provide about the very highest levels of cerebral function. Even if we cannot explain why the distributions are as they are, they provide an objective way of seeing whether behaviour has significantly improved, deteriorated, or remained essentially the same. They may also suggest the nature of the underlying dysfunction.

However, a snag with saccadometry is that it is idiosyncratic. As we saw in Figure 2.9, Chapter 2, although two or three parameters are all we need to summarise the performance of a single subject, and in the absence of disease these parameters remain stable over time, they vary greatly from one person to another. This has two consequences. First, a single measurement in one patient is essentially meaningless, unless it is grossly different from the norm (or if there is left/right difference). What is essential is to use longitudinal studies, with one distribution measured before the injury or treatment and the other after; and preferably, of course, more measurements in the follow-up period. The second consequence is that comparisons of populations tend to be weak, since the idiosyncrasies greatly increase the variance of measures across the population. However, to compensate, the equipment and protocols lend themselves to international standardisation, effectively increasing the size of the populations being compared (Antoniades, Ettinger et al. 2013).

In this Appendix we skim briefly over some examples of using saccadometry more or less successfully in providing quantitative measures of higher cerebral function. Much more thorough accounts, with wider scope, can be found in, for example, Leigh and Kennard (2004), and Leigh and Zee (2015).

App 2.1 Degenerative Conditions

App 2.1.1 Parkinson's Disease

Michell, Xu et al. (2006), Perneczky, Ghosh et al. (2011) – L-dopa was found to increase saccadic latency of Parkinson's disease (PD) patients, and this could be modelled by an increased threshold in the LATER model. Higher μ (shorter latency) was positively correlated with grey matter volume of the prefrontal cortex and cerebellar vermis in PD patients (Perneczky, Ghosh et al. 2011).

Antoniades, Xu et al. (2013) – Saccadic latency and manual (hand) response latency are both similarly increased in PD compared with normal control subjects, reflecting a similar increase in μ.

App 2.1.2 Deep Brain Stimulation

Temel, Visser-Vandewalle et al. (2008) – In PD patients with deep brain stimulators (DBS) inserted in the subthalamic nuclei, bilateral electrical stimulation led to an increased saccadic latency that corresponded to an increased μ in the LATER model. This implies that DBS enhances the gain of the descending basal ganglia pathways that initiate saccades. It has subsequently been shown that this improvement in response times also applies to manual responses implying a more general effect not limited to saccades (Antoniades, Carpenter et al. 2012). Note that insertion of the stimulators themselves gives a transient increase of saccadic latency prior to this improvement (Antoniades, Buttery et al. 2012).

App 2.1.3 Huntington's Disease

Ali, Michell et al. (2006) – The use of saccadometry in patients with Huntington's disease (HD) revealed these patients have increased latency and more early saccades compared with normal subjects, and parameterising these differences was sensitive enough to diagnose HD patients (Antoniades, Altham et al. 2007). Monitoring of HD patients over three years from prior to disease manifestation to established disease revealed a clear progression of saccadic abnormalities, suggesting that studying these eye movements may help track disease progression (Robert, Nachev et al. 2009, Antoniades, Zheyu et al. 2010). It is thought that there are two parallel paths descending from frontal cortex to substantia nigra pars reticulata, which then inhibits the colliculus: an indirect tonically inhibitory one via GPe and the subthalamus, and an excitatory one going directly from the caudate and putamen to SNpr; in HD the indirect pathway is impaired, leading to an increase in spontaneous, unsuppressed, movement (Peitsch, Hoffman et al. 2008) and giving longer saccadic latencies.

App 2.1.4 Progressive Supranuclear Palsy

Antoniades, Bak et al. (2007) – Analysing saccadic latency distributions revealed that progressive supranuclear palsy (PSP) patients can be discriminated from patients with other parkinsonian conditions based on parameters of LATER modelling of these distributions, suggesting saccadometry may be a useful diagnostic tool here.

Ghosh, Carpenter et al. (2013) – Saccadic abnormalities in PSP patients progress at different rates compared with other motor and cognitive deficits, likely reflecting differential deterioration in their underlying cortical–subcortical circuits.

App 2.1.5 Amyotrophic Lateral Sclerosis

Burrell, Carpenter et al. (2013) – Measuring saccadic latencies in amyotrophic lateral sclerosis (ALS) patients revealed a higher number of early saccades compared with normal subjects, but all other saccadic parameters were normal.

App 2.1.6 Dementia

Burrell, Hornberger et al. (2012) – The use of saccadometry in patients with frontotemporal dementia (FTD) demonstrated an increase in early saccades and also the saccadic latency, corresponding with reduced μ, compared with normal subjects. These deficits were correlated with atrophy of the left frontal eye field in these patients, as determined by brain imaging. Other work has similarly showed that FTD patients have impaired ability to withhold an antisaccade (Meyniel, Rivaud-Péchoux et al. 2005).

App 2.2 General Neurology

App 2.2.1 Anaesthetics

Nouraei, de Pennington et al. (2003) – In human subjects being administered the general anaesthetic sevofluorane, increasing doses of drug led to increased saccadic

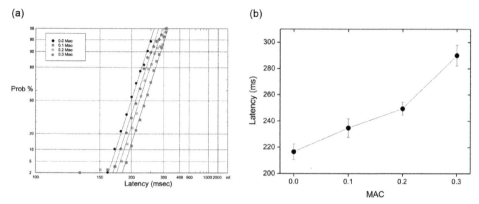

Figure App 2.1 Effect of different levels of sevofluorane sedation. (a) Higher sedation levels are associated with longer latencies. (b) Dose-response relationships, average of 5 subjects. 1 MAC represents the minimum average anaesthetic dose (Nouraei, de Pennington et al. 2003).

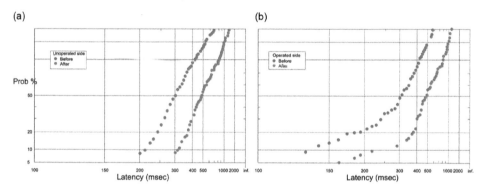

Figure App 2.2 Saccadic latency distributions on the unoperated (a) and operated (b) side before and after a stroke brought on by carotid endarterectomy. Note the very large increase in median latency on both sides, and the larger number of early response on the operated side both before and after the operation (Nouraei, Roos et al. 2010).

latency as well as stop signal reaction times in a countermanding task, suggesting saccadic measurements could be used to estimate the cortical effects of general anaesthetics (Khan, Taylor et al. 1999), Figure App 2.1.

App 2.2.2 Endarterectomy

Endarterectomy and other vascular surgery affecting the blood supply to the brain can often be followed by cerebral deterioration or even stroke because of blocking of small blood vessels by dislodged debris (Walsh, Nouraei et al.

2010). In general, deleterious effects are more marked on the operated side (Nouraei, Roos et al. 2010) , but so are the benefits from improved cerebral perfusion (Figure App 2.2). This is a good example of left–right differences in latency providing more useful information than can be generated, for example, by paper-and-pencil 'cognitive' tests.

App 2.2.3 Migraine

Measurements of saccades in patients with migraine (although not having migraine episodes at the time) showed

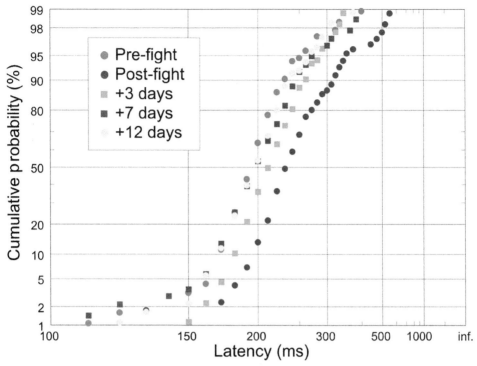

Figure App 2.3 Reversible effect of mild traumatic brain injury. Latencies for a saccadic step task just before a boxing match (red), immediately after (blue), and at various times thereafter. The subject showed signs of mild concussion during the bout, reflected in the increased latency after it; but over 12 days' time, the distribution gradually returned to normal (Pearson, Armitage et al. 2007).

these patients have reduced variability in reaction times compared with normal subjects, pointing towards a functional deficit in noradrenergic systems influencing the cerebral cortex (Chandna, Chandrasekharan et al. 2012). Moreover, patients with more severe migraines produced more anti-saccade errors, implying a deficit in inhibitory control processes.

App 2.2.4 Traumatic Brain Injury

Another potential field of application is in evaluating concussion (mild traumatic brain injury) – an area that has recently become the focus of much public concern, particularly in contact sports such as football, in horse-riding, and in military personnel (Putukian, Echemendia et al. 2000). In all these cases, the value of the

test can be greatly enhanced by making baseline measurements in advance, so that responses can be tracked in the same person, rather than relying on group statistics. Preliminary work has been encouraging in suggesting that while blows to the head may create quite substantial shifts of the distribution to longer latencies, these appear to revert to normal over a matter of days (Figure App 2.3) (Pearson, Armitage et al. 2007).

App 2.2.5 Hepatic Encephalopathy

Patients with liver cirrhosis develop hepatic encephalopathy, which is typically assessed only subjectively and therefore is difficult to quantify (Krismer, Roos et al. 2010). In patients with hepatic encephalopathy due to liver cirrhosis, measurements of saccades revealed that there were prolonged saccadic latencies compared with normal control subjects, providing a potentially quantitative means of assessing hepatic encephalopathy. These findings were subsequently extended to covert hepatic encephalopathy (a more subtle cognitive deficit) in liver cirrhosis patients (Cunniffe, Munby et al. 2015).

App 2.3 Miscellaneous

App 2.3.1 Psychiatric Disorders

Saccadic deficits have been identified in psychiatric patients. For example, schizophrenia patients perform poorly (producing more errors, for example) in the antisaccade task compared with normal subjects, as do a high proportion of non-psychotic first-degree relatives of schizophrenia patients (McDowell, Myles-Worsley et al. 1999, Broerse, Crawford et al. 2001, Reuter and Kathmann 2004, Cutsuridis, Kumari et al. 2014). Similarly, schizophrenia patients also produce more errors and fewer correction responses in a double-step (Wheeless) task (Thakkar, Schall et al. 2015). Saccadometry is now being recognised as a promising tool for exploring cognitive deficits in psychiatric disorders (Hutton and Ettinger 2006, Smyrnis 2008).

App 2.3.2 Metabolic

Dawson, Murphy et al. (2011) – Patients with phenylketoneurea (PKU) who are untreated (i.e., not on a protein-restricted diet) develop cognitive deficits, which may be difficult to quantify or even detect. Measuring saccades in PKU patients not on a protein-restricted diet showed these patients had slower reaction times than normal controls and PKU patients on a diet.

App 2.3.3 Storage Diseases

Roos, Lachmann et al. (2006) – Saccade latencies were significantly prolonged in patients with Sandhoff disease compared with normal subjects, and this correlated with performance in tests of motor function, indicating that saccade latency is a clinically relevant parameter in this disease.

App 2.3.4 Ageing

Measuring saccade latencies in subjects of different age groups performing antisaccades showed that young children had slow reaction times and the most errors, young adults had shorter reaction times, and older adults had slower reaction times (Munoz, Broughton et al. 1998). These results reveal the effects of brain development and degeneration on oculomotor performance (Figure App 2.4).

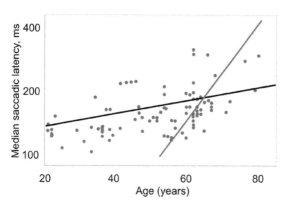

Figure App 2.4 Median saccadic latency as a function of age in 90 normal controls. The black line has a slope of 1 ms per year, the blue line of 10 ms per year. This difference may perhaps reflect increasing impairment of cerebral blood supply in older people. (R. H. S. Carpenter, unpublished data).

Appendix 3 Practical

To me this small dark room, cluttered with apparatus and a tangle of wires, is a place of infinite possibilities and far horizons, full of pathways looking into the unknown
Kenneth Craik, The Nature of Explanation *(1952)*

App 3.1 Measuring Saccadic Latency Distributions

'Eye trackers' are popular items in cognitive scientists' grant proposals. But when eventually one sees the Methods section of the resultant papers, it is clear that rather few know what they're for or understand their technical limitations. They are particularly unsuitable for making measurements of latency distributions. What they measure is *gaze*: the direction of the line of sight relative to the outside world (see Chapter 1, Section 1.1). It therefore depends on head position, which has to be taken into account by the eye tracker, often by having short calibration sessions at intervals during the experiment. To save time, these are often simply 9-point calibrations, which deal with any shifts or simple rescalings caused by head movement, but do not deal with non-linearities and disrupt the experimental run. These problems can be greatly reduced by using a bite-bar (ideally), or at least a headrest; otherwise, they contribute substantially to the device's inaccuracy.

A virtue of the ordinary eye-tracker is that it measures vertical as well as horizontal eye movements, and is also capable of measuring vergence. Portable versions now exist, often mounted on spectacle frames, but are not good at sensing head position. Consequently, eye-trackers are usually set up in laboratories, which

is inconvenient from a clinical point of view.

The *saccadometer*, on the other hand, is much less versatile and designed for a very specific task – the measurement of saccadic latency, in response to visual stimuli it generates for itself. It is essentially a self-contained device, but its output can be sent in real time to a computer that runs an experiment by presenting the subject with more-or-less complex and programmable protocols, measuring eye position as well as latency. In this mode, it is convenient to call it an *oculometer* rather than saccadometer.

App 3.2 Recording

App 3.2.1 The Saccadometer

The saccadometer is a highly specialised medical and research instrument that automatically measures and analyses the latencies and durations of large numbers of saccades, evoked by visual stimuli generated by laser projectors mounted on the device itself (Ober, Przedpelska-Ober et al. 2003). It measures eye movements by means of direct infrared (IR) oculography and is optimised for easy set up and minimal intrusiveness, which are crucial for monitoring oculomotor function in a non-laboratory setting. It is non-invasive and self-contained: the transducer (Figure App 3.1) is connected to a small controller box that generates the stimuli and stores the resultant eye movements. Many sessions can be stored and then downloaded to a computer. It is self-calibrating, normally done at the beginning of a session and taking a matter of seconds. Once started, an experiment can be left to run by itself. As a result, it is possible to run several sessions

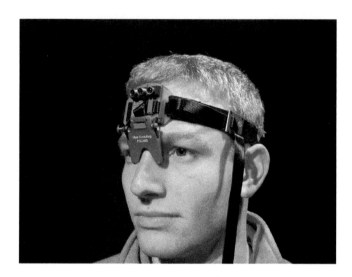

Figure App 3.1 A subject wearing a saccadometer. At the top, three lasers project visual targets that move with the head. The eye-movement transducer rests on the nose, and therefore also moves with the head. The device is connected to a stand-alone control box that stores data which can be downloaded later.

in parallel, for instance, in a changing room after a sporting event.

It does not require any kind of mechanical adjustments of the sensor position in relation to the eye, thus saving a great deal of time and enabling measurements to be performed by relatively untrained personnel: all necessary adjustments are performed automatically by the saccadometer control system.

App 3.2.2 The Oculometer

The oculometer uses exactly the same transducer as the saccadometer, but generates a voltage proportional to eye position that can be sent to a computer via an analog-to-digital converter. The computer can then generate complex protocols using relatively sophisticated stimuli, such as RDKs (Chapter 4, Section 4.6.1).

Unlike other IR oculography systems, which require the infrared emitters/sensors to be placed around the eye in its direct vicinity, the transducers are located between the eyes, thus hiding the sensor assembly behind the 'shadow' of the nose. This arrangement does not limit the visual field, and the measuring system can work without interfering with the subject's visual functions. The inner canthi of the

left and right eyes are illuminated with low-intensity IR light, and any differences between the amounts reflected back from the eye surfaces carry information about eye position changes. The bandwidth is 250 Hz, with a noise level equivalent to 0.1 degree.

The measuring range (along the horizontal axis) is ±35 deg. The calculated value of non-linearity is 2% on average and 4.5% in the worst case, giving 0.4 deg and 0.9 deg, respectively (Figure App 3.2). Of course, from the point of view of measuring both latency and duration, linearity is essentially irrelevant.

The voltage generated by the electromagnetic (EM) sensor is digitised into 12-bit data at a sampling rate of 1 kHz and afterwards differentiated to create an eye velocity signal. Saccades are identified as the instances when the eye velocity exceeds a velocity threshold of 5 deg/s.

App 3.2.3 Using the Saccadometer for Manual Responses

The saccadometer control unit has three light-emitting diodes (LEDs) and corresponding push buttons for making manual responses. Normally, the LEDs are turned on and off in synchrony with the lasers,

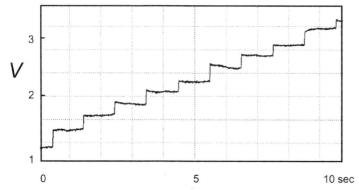

Figure App 3.2 Saccadometer output (volts) from one subject making saccades to 10 targets spaced 2 deg apart (courtesy Professor Jan Ober).

and the buttons generate signals that are interpreted by the system as being saccades. Using SPIC (Saccadic Peak Velocity and Impulse Computer) software, the LEDs and buttons can be programmed as flexibly as needed.

App 3.3 Generating Visual Stimuli

App 3.3.1 Saccadometer

An important feature of the saccadometer is that it generates its own stimuli, using lasers attached to the transducer that therefore move with the head. This means that there is no need to immobilise the head, and subjects can sit comfortably. The lasers would normally project on to some convenient surface a meter or so away. This distance does not matter much, since in angular terms the subtense of the lines of projection will be constant. Therefore, it is not essential for a subject's refractive error to be corrected by spectacles: they can choose whatever distance gives best vision. In a clinical setting, the patient can lie on a bed and project the targets on the ceiling. It is not normally necessary to adjust the brightness of the background, as the small spots generated by the lasers have extremely high intensity, and contrast is therefore very high and beyond the range at which it

contributes significantly to latency (Chapter 4, Section 4.7).

App 3.3.2 Oculometer

The oculometer relies on exact synchronisation between the moment of generating the response and the start of the eye movement record. In general, this is impossible to achieve without special precautions: the computer's operating system may disregard incoming information because it is busy with something else, and an ordinary display system can behave autonomously, deciding the moment to update different parts of the display. Experimenters should also be aware of interleaving of the display and that a frame starts to be displayed at the top, so that with a 100 Hz frame rate, and allowing for interleaving, the lower parts will be delayed by some 20 ms. In general, all this means for the purpose of measuring saccadic latency is that very high frame and sampling rates are completely pointless; overall sampling at 100 Hz is perfectly adequate, both from a technical point of view and in terms of how to present the resultant distributions.

Finally, compared with cathode-ray tubes (CRTs), modern flat-screen displays are extremely non-uniform, in the sense that brightness is a function of viewing angle: this can, for instance, result in colours changing when the subject's head moves. However, though CRTs are now effectively obsolete, some progress is being made on alternative display systems. Some of these issues are discussed in Carpenter and Robson (1998), including the specific problems posed by colour (Mollon and Baker 1995).

App 3.3.3 ViSaGe and SPIC

The system we currently use for recording and analysing saccadic latency is called SPIC (Carpenter 1994). In real-time experiments, it uses the more versatile display facilities provided by systems such as the ViSaGe (Visual Stimulus Generator and Analyser) from Cambridge Research Systems, with its high frame rate synchronised to the recording of eye movements, but also analyses data that have previously been obtained from a saccadometer. It provides a simple language for creating quite complex sequences of visual and auditory stimuli, using the ViSaGe, as well as the software for recording and analysing saccades and their latencies, including estimation of LATER parameters. It also enables the user to create simulations of complex decision systems and test them directly against observations. SPIC can be downloaded free from the Web, and has a very comprehensive help file, describing file formats and the details of how to generate complex protocols and stimuli.

App 3.4 Protocol Design

App 3.4.1 Interleaving

Because the oculomotor system is so good at spotting any kind of predictability in the presentation of stimuli, one needs to be particularly careful to try to avoid trial-by-trial regularities in the choice of stimuli. For a simple step task, this means that the direction of each trial should be selected independently of that of the previous trial. But this does not mean having exactly half the trials in one direction and the other half in the other, as it may happen by chance that towards the end of the run we may end up with a preponderance of whichever direction previously happened to occur less often, a point touched on in Section 6.2.1 in Chapter 6. As far as the saccadometer is concerned, one must choose from a fixed repertoire of possible protocols, which can include the step task, appearance and gap, and antisaccades, and the random interleaving is implemented automatically. Using SPIC, extremely complex protocols and stimuli can be programmed using the built-in descriptive languages, so one can specify any interleaving in some detail.

App 3.4.2 Speeding Things Up

Experiments using either the saccadometer or oculometer can be performed very fast. For the simplest tasks, such as step responses, it is not difficult to record some 20 to 30 trials in a minute. Generally, the higher the rate, the better it is for the subject, partly to reduce boredom or fatigue, and also partly to prevent the subject from thinking too much about the task and how well they are performing. The latter can be extremely important in a clinical situation, where the patient may be genuinely anxious about their performance, for instance, in antisaccade tasks where they will be aware of their errors.

So we need the shortest inter-trial times that still allow the subject time to re-fixate centrally without feeling rushed, combined with foreperiods – ideally non-ageing (see Chapter 4, Section 4.2.1) – that are on average something like 500 ms in duration.

App 3.4.3 Alertness

With longer runs, the subject is inevitably going to find it difficult not to become bored or drowsy. This can often generate a number of 'late' responses (see Chapter 2, Section 2.2.2), or even failure to respond at all. It's then probably a good idea to have a break, though simply making a noise is often sufficient to get them back on track. Simply talking to them may be sufficient to keep them at a relatively steady level of arousal (experiments show that this has surprisingly little effect on their performance, provided they're not expected to reply). In addition, it is helpful to introduce short breaks of a minute or so at regular intervals, with drinks or snacks if desired. It is better not to tell subjects that this is about to happen, or how many trials remain in the run as a whole, as this is likely to influence their alertness, and they may start mentally ticking off how many remain to do.

App 3.4.4 How Many Trials?

This is obviously related to alertness. It is unreasonable – and counter-productive – to expect a subject to be able to perform in a consistent way over more than an hour – say, up to 1000 trials or so. But with half-hour breaks in between, most subjects can manage say three one-hour sessions in an afternoon without undue fatigue.

To establish the main parameters, 100 data points are usually plenty; to make precise estimates of particular features of the shape (for instance, to distinguish swivel from shift) usually requires something more like 1000. This may sound daunting, but with computer-controlled automatic systems like SPIC and the saccadometer, a trial in a simple experiment like the step task lasts some 3 seconds. So, 1000 trials need not occupy much more than an hour, even with a few breaks. Bear in mind also that for some tasks (countermanding, Go / NoGo) a certain proportion of the trials necessarily generate no data, and this must be taken into account. In addition, a certain proportion of trials will always have to be

rejected because the saccadic trajectory is malformed; experience shows that this less true of well-practised subjects. 'Malformed' here means not starting at the central fixation point, or finishing at the intended end-point, or perturbed by noise of one kind or another, for example, through eyelid movement. These are to a large extent eliminated automatically by the saccadometer, but not by the oculometer, and should always be checked trial by trial. Responses that are impossibly fast (for example, occurring before the stimulus) should be eliminated at the same time.

App 3.4.5 Standardisation

One of the virtues of the saccadometer is that though deployed by many groups worldwide, its stimuli and protocols are standardised. This makes it very easy to compare or even combine results from different groups, which is particularly important in the clinical field and especially with rare conditions. In the case of antisaccades, a standard protocol has been published that facilitates this kind of comparison (Antoniades, Ettinger et al. 2013).

App 3.5 Analysing Distributions

Statistics do not make subjective judgements objective; they simply substitute one kind of subjectiveness for another, generally by simplifying the data, and by making assumptions. If the results are already self-evident – perhaps a piece of litmus that is red when others are blue, or a leaden ball and wooden ball that drop in equal times from a tower – to measure variances and calculate significance levels is superfluous.

To p or not to p is a frequent cause of culture-clash between physiologists and psychologists. Psychologists love statistics, being trained to believe nothing that has not some kind of $p = x\%$ attached to it, and to be adept in conjuring silk purses out of pigs' ears; physiologists loathe stats and do them only *in extremis*, when the data are so appalling that there is some actual doubt about whether they means anything at all. Someone who has trained in both disciplines will probably prefer a pragmatic approach adapted to circumstances.

In any case, what we are analysing here are *distributions*, which have their statistics already built into them. To show histograms is to provide far more information about the statistics of the underlying process than would be conveyed by summary measures like mean reaction time and its variance or other moments. It also obliges the experimenter actually to think about the results. Over the past decade or so there has been a regrettable tendency for the 'Results' section of a typical paper to consist entirely of a list of 'effects' that have clearly been generated automatically by an ANOVA sausage-machine, without passing through a human mind. It shouldn't be necessary to emphasise the need to frame some hypothesis before examining the observed data and ask yourself specifically whether the data do or do not support that hypothesis.

There are four main kinds of questions one may want to ask about distributions:

1. What is the probability that one observed distribution is generated by the same stochastic process as another?

2. What is the probability that an observed distribution could have been generated by a given theoretical model (for instance, LATER)?

3. Does an observed distribution fit one model better than another?

4. Is there a significant difference between responses to the right and left?

For (1), (2), and (4), the best test is probably the Kolmogorov–Smirnov (KS) (Kolmogorov 1941, Smirnov 1948) . It is a non-parametric test that makes no assumptions about the underlying forms of the distributions: the one-sample KS test deals with (2), and the two-sample test with (1) and (4). For (3), we tend to use likelihood tests, which make no assumptions beyond what are built in to the models, and have the advantage that log likelihood ratios for alternative hypotheses simply sum across subjects

Do left/right differences in control trials matter? Most published studies ignore them unless they are very large, and it is true to say that in many cases they tend to come and go, possibly as a result of experiencing different stimuli from the outside world, but are also more marked at the start of a run. In general, differences of up to 20 ms are probably meaningless, and in any case – unless the number of trials is large – may not be significant as far as KS is concerned. If two distributions are not significantly different, then one is fully justified in combining them. On the other hand, significant left/right differences may also be an important sign of unilateral impairment, especially if we are fortunate enough to have data collected before and after some critical event such as traumatic brain injury, a stroke, or a clinical intervention of some kind (see, for example, Figure App 2.2 in Appendix 2).

3.5.1 How to Create a Reciprobit Plot

There are various ways of generating reciprobit plots.

1. Use SPIC. Prepare your raw histogram as a text file, which should consist of a series of lines each of the form <lat> <n>, where <lat> is the lower bound of a latency bin of 10 msec width, and <n> is the number of responses in the bin; they are separated by a space or

tab. Give the file the extension .LAR, and read it in SPIC. This method provides good-quality graphics, and allows you to use SPIC's full analytical power. If you have something like a ViSaGe system, then the data will be automatically imported at the end of a run. Or if your data have been generated by a saccadometer, they can be downloaded directly into SPIC for further (offline) analysis.

2. Use Excel, or a data-plotting application such as SigmaPlot or Origin. They may allow you to set up the required reciprocal and probit axes, but you will have to generate cumulative histograms. In Excel, you need to make the transforms explicit (use the NORMSINV function for the probit scale). All of this can be a lot of work and is already done for you by SPIC. Why re-invent the wheel?

3. A legacy technique, but quite satisfying, is to draw the graph by hand on the special reciprobit paper, which can be downloaded from the SPIC website. It won't, of course, do any analysis for you, but the shear act of drawing graphs by hand can surprisingly often generate insights that a more automated system will hide from you.

Bibliography

Aantaa, E., P. J. Riekkinen and H. J. Frey (1973). "Electronystagmographic findings in multiple sclerosis." *Acta Otolaryngologica* **75**: 1–5.

Abadi, R. V., D. S. Broomhead, R. A. Clement, J. P. Whittle and R. Worfolk (1997). "Dynamical systems analysis: a new method of analysing congenital nystagmus waveforms." *Experimental Brain Research* **117**: 355–361.

Adams, M. W. J., D. Wood and R. H. S. Carpenter (2000). "Expectation acuity: the spatial specificity of the effect of prior probability on saccadic latency." *Journal of Physiology* **527**(**P**): 140–141.

Aizawa, H., R. Amo and H. Okamoto (2011). "Phylogeny and ontogeny of the habenular structure." *Frontiers in Neuroscience* **5**: 2–7.

Ali, F. R., A. W. Michell, R. A. Barker and R. H. S. Carpenter (2006). "The use of quantitative oculometry in the assessment of Huntington's disease." *Experimental Brain Research* **169**: 237–245.

Anderson, A. J. and R. H. S. Carpenter (2004). "Dynamics of probability prediction in a saccadic latency task." *Journal of Physiology*: 555P D554.

Anderson, A. J. and R. H. S. Carpenter (2006). "Changes in expectation consequent on experience, modelled by a simple, forgetful neural circuit." *Journal of Vision* **6**: 822–835.

Anderson, A. J. and R. H. S. Carpenter (2010). "Saccadic latency in deterministic environments: getting back on track after the unexpected happens." *Journal of Vision* **10:14**: 12.

Anderson, A. J., H. Yadav and R. H. S. Carpenter (2008). "Directional prediction by the saccadic system." *Current Biology* **18**: 614–618.

Anderson, J. A. (1993). The BSB model: a simple nonlinear autoassociative neural network. *Associative Neural Networks: Theory and Implementation*. M. H. Hassoun, ed. Oxford, Oxford University Press: 77–103.

Antoniades, C., U. Ettinger, B. Gaymard, et al. (2013). "An internationally standardized antisaccade protocol for clinical use." *Vision Research* **84**: 1–5.

Antoniades, C. A., P. M. E. Altham, S. L. Mason, R. A. Barker and R. H. S. Carpenter (2007). "Saccadometry: a new tool for evaluating pre-symptomatic Huntington patients." *Neuroreport* **18**: 1133–1136.

Antoniades, C. A., T. H. Bak, R. H. S. Carpenter, J. H. Hodges and R. A. Barker (2007). "The diagnostic potential of saccadometry in progressive supranuclear palsy." *Biomarkers in Medicine* **1**: 487–490.

Antoniades, C. A., P. Buttery, J. F. FitzGerald, et al. (2012). "Deep brain stimulation: eye movements reveal anomalous effects of electrode placement and stimulation." *PLoS ONE* **7**: e32830.

Antoniades, C. A. and R. H. S. Carpenter (2012). "Making neurology quantitative." *Neuroreport* **23**: 572–575.

Antoniades, C. A., R. H. S. Carpenter and Y. Temel (2012). "Deep brain stimulation of the subthalamic nucleus in Parkinson's disease: similar improvements in saccadic and manual responses." *Neuroreport* **23**: 179–183.

Antoniades, C. A., Z. Xu, R. H. Carpenter and R. A. Barker (2013). "The relationship between abnormalities of saccadic and manual response times in Parkinson's disease." *Journal of Parkinson's Disease* **3**: 557–563.

Antoniades, C. A., X. Zheyu, S. L. Mason, R. H. S. Carpenter and R. A. Barker (2010). "Huntington's disease: changes in saccades and hand-tapping over three years." *Journal of Neurology* **257**: 1890–1898.

Aron, A. R., P. C. Fletcher, E. T. Bullmore, B. J. Sahakian and T. W. Robbins (2003).

"Stop-signal inhibition disrupted by damage to right inferior frontal gyrus in humans." *Nature Neuroscience* **6**: 115–116.

Aron, A. R., B. J. Sahakian and T. W. Robbins (2003). "Distractibility during selection for action: differential deficits in Huntington s disease and following frontal lobe damage." *Neuropsychologia* **41**: 1137–1147.

Aron, A. R., F. Schlagheeken, P. C. Fletcher, et al. (2002). "Inhibition of subliminally primed responses is mediated by the caudate and thalamus: evidence from functional MRI and Huntington's disease." *Brain* **126**: 713–723.

Asimov, I. (1984). *New Guide to Science*. New York, Basic Books.

Asrress, K. N. and R. H. S. Carpenter (2001). "Saccadic countermanding: a comparison of central and peripheral stop signals." *Vision Research* **41**: 2645–2651.

Audley, R. J. (1960). "A stochastic model for individual choice behaviour." *Psychological Review* **67**: 1–15.

Avila, A. and S.-C. Lin (2014). "Motivational salience signal in the basal forebrain is coupled with faster and more precise decision speed." *PLOS Biology* **12**(3): 1–13.

Babbage, Charles. (1989) "Letter to Sir David Brewster, LLD., on the subject of Mr. Babbage's Calculating Engines." *The Works of Charles Babbage*. M. Campbell-Kelly, ed. London, Pickering and Chatto: 77.

Bacon, F. (1605). *The Advancement of Learning*. London, Pickering.

Balfour, A. J. (1914). *Theism and Humanism*. New York, Hodder and Stoughton.

Baraclough, D. J., M. I. Conroy and D. Lee (2004). "Prefrontal cortex and decision making in a mixed-strategy game." *Nature Neuroscience* **7**: 404–410.

Barlow, H. (1990). "Conditions for versatile learning, Helmholtz's unconscious inference, and the task of perception." *Vision Research* **30**: 1561–1571.

Barlow, H. and S. P. Tripathy (1997). "Correspondence noise and signal pooling in the detection of coherent visual motion." *Journal of Neuroscience* **17**: 7954–7966.

Barlow, H. B. (1957). "Increment thresholds at low intensities considered as signal/noise discriminations." *Journal of Physiology* **136**: 469–488.

Barlow, H. B. (1980). "The absolute efficiency of perceptual decisions." *Philosophical Transactions of the Royal Society* **290**: 71–82.

Barlow, H. B., A. M. Derrington, L. R. Harris and P. Lennie (1977). "The effects of remote stimulation on the responses of cat retinal ganglion cells." *Journal of Physiology* **269**: 177–194.

Bartlett, F. C. (1932). *Remembering: A Study in Experimental and Social Psychology*. Cambridge, Cambridge University Press.

Bass, T. (1991). *The Newtonian Casino*. London, Penguin Press.

Basso, M. A. and R. H. Wurtz (1998). "Modulation of neuronal activity in superior colliculus by changes in target probability." *Journal of Neuroscience* **18**(18): 7519–7534.

Bayes, T. (1763). "Essay toward solving a problem in the doctrine of chances." *Philosophical Transactions of the Royal Society* **53**: 370–418.

Beck, J. M., W. J. Ma, R. Kiani, et al. (2008). "Probabilistic population codes for Bayesian decision making." *Neuron* **60**: 1142–1152.

Becker, W. and R. Jürgens (1975). Saccadic reactions to double-step stimuli: evidence for model feedback and continuous information uptake. *Basic Mechanisms of Ocular Motility and Their Clinical Implications*. G. Lennerstrand and P. Bach-y-Rita, eds. Oxford, Pergamon: 519–524.

Becker, W. and R. Jürgens (1979). "An analysis of the saccadic system by means of double-step stimuli." *Vision Research* **19**: 967–983.

Beintema, J., E. M. van Loon, I. T. C. Hooge and A. van der Berg (2003). "Saccadic decision-rate distributions reveal competitive process." *Journal of Vision* **3**: 72a.

Berg, H. C. and D. A. Brown (1972). "Chemotaxis in *Escherichia coli* analysed by three-dimensional tracking." *Nature* **239**: 500–504.

Bianco, I. H. and S. W. Wilson (2009). "The habenular nuclei: a conserved asymmetric relay station in the vertebrate brain." *Philosophical Transaction of the Royal Society B* **364**: 1005–1020.

Bloch, M. A. M. (1885). "Expériences sur la vision." *Comptes rendus des séances de la Société de Biologie et de ses filiales* **2**: 493–495.

Boring, E. G. (1929). *A History of Experimental Psychology.* New York, Century.

Boucher, L., T. J. Palmieri, G. D. Logan and J. D. Schall (2007). "Inhibitory control in mind and brain: an interactive race model of countermanding saccades." *Psychological Review* **114**: 376–397.

Bray, D. (2009). *Wetware: A Computer in Every Living Cell.* New Haven, Yale University Press.

Bray, T. J. P. and R. H. S. Carpenter (2015). "Saccadic foraging: reduced reaction time to informative targets." *European Journal of Neuroscience* **41**: 908–913.

Brockman, D. and T. Geisel (1999). "Are human scanpaths Lévy flights?" *Ninth International Conference on Artificial Neural Networks: ICANN 99* (Conf. Publ. No. 470). Edinburgh: 263–268, vol. 1.

Brockman, D. and T. Geisel (2000). "The ecology of gaze shifts." *Neurocomputing* **32**: 643–650.

Brodersen, K. H., W. D. Penny, L. M. Harrison, et al. (2008). "Integrated Bayesian models of learning and decision making for saccadic eye movements." *Neural Networks* **21**: 1247–1260.

Broerse, A., T. J. Crawford and J. A. den Boer (2001). "Parsing cognition in schizophrenia using saccadic eye movements: a selective overview." *Neuropsychologia* **39**: 742–756.

Brown, H. D. and A. Heathcote (2008). "The simplest complete model of choice response time: linear ballistic accumulation." *Cognitive Psychology* **57**: 153–178.

Brown, J. W. (2014). "The tale of the neuroscientists and the computer: why mechanistic theory matters." *Frontiers in Neuroscience* **8**: 1–3.

Brown, P., C. C. Chen, S. Wang, et al. (2006). "Involvement of human basal ganglia in offline feedback control of voluntary movement." *Current Biology* **16**: 2129–2134.

Burrell, J. R., R. H. S. Carpenter, J. R. Hodges and M. C. Kiernan (2013). "Early saccades in amyotrophic lateral sclerosis." *Amyotrophic Lateral Sclerosis and Frontotemporal Degeneration* **14**: 294–301.

Burrell, J. R., M. Hornberger, R. H. S. Carpenter, M. C. Kiernan and J. R. Hodges (2012). "Saccadic abnormalities in frontotemporal dementia." *Neurology* **78**: 1816–1823.

Camalier, C. R., A. Gotier, A. Murthy, et al. (2007). "Dynamics of saccade target selection: race model analysis of double step and search step saccade production in human and macaque." *Vision Research* **47**: 2187–2211.

Campbell, F. W. and J. J. Kulikowski (1972). "The visual evoked potential as a function of contrast of a grating pattern." *Journal of Physiology* **222**: 345–356.

Carpenter, R. (2000). "The neural control of looking." *Current Biology* **10**(8): R291–293.

Carpenter, R. and I. Noorani (2017). "Movement suppression: brain mechanisms for stopping and stillness." *Philosophical Transaction of the Royal Society B: Biological Sciences* **372**(1718).

Carpenter, R. and B. Reddi (2012). *Neurophysiology: A Conceptual Approach.* London, Hodder.

Carpenter, R. H. S. (1981). Oculomotor procrastination. *Eye Movements: Cognition and Visual Perception.* D. F. Fisher, R. A. Monty and J. W. Senders, eds. Hillsdale, Lawrence Erlbaum: 237–246.

Carpenter, R. H. S. (1988). *Movements of the Eyes.* London, Pion.

Carpenter, R. H. S., ed. (1992a). *Eye Movements.* Vol. 8, *Vision and Visual Dysfunction.* London, Macmillan.

Carpenter, R. H. S. (1992b). The visual origins of ocular motility. *Eye Movements.* Vol. 8,

Vision and Visual Dysfunction. R. H. S. Carpenter, ed. London, Macmillan: 1–10.

Carpenter, R. H. S. (1993). "The distribution of quick phase intervals in optokinetic nystagmus." *Ophthalmic Research* **25**: 91–93.

Carpenter, R. H. S. (1994). Express optokinetic nystagmus. *Contemporary Ocular Motor and Vestibular Research.* A. F. Fuchs, T. Brandt, U. Büttner and D. Zee, eds. Stuttgart, Georg Thieme: 185–187.

Carpenter, R. H. S. (1994). "Frontal cortex: choosing where to look." *Current Biology* **4**: 341–343.

Carpenter, R. H. S. (1994). "SPIC: a PC-based system for rapid measurement of saccadic responses." *Journal of Physiology (Proceedings)* **480**: 4P.

Carpenter, R. H. S. (2001). "Express saccades: is bimodality a result of the order of stimulus presentation?" *Vision Research* **41**: 1145–1151.

Carpenter, R. H. S. (2004). "The saccadic system: a neurological microcosm." *Advances in Clinical Neuroscience and Rehabilitation* **4**: 6–8.

Carpenter, R. H. S. (2004). "Supplementary eye field: keeping an eye on eye movement." *Current Biology* **14**: R416–418.

Carpenter, R. H. S. (2012). "Analysing the detail of saccadic reaction time distributions." *Biocybernetics and Biological Engineering* **32**: 49–63.

Carpenter, R. H. S. and V. Kinsler (1995). "Saccadic eye movements while reading music." *Vision Research* **35**: 1447–1458.

Carpenter, R. H. S. and S. A. McDonald (2006). "LATER predicts saccade latency distributions in reading." *Experimental Brain Research* **177**: 176–183.

Carpenter, R. H. S. and B. A. J. Reddi (2001). "Deciding between the deciders: two models of reaction time may happily coexist." *Nature Neuroscience* **4**: 337.

Carpenter, R. H. S., B. A. J. Reddi and A. J. Anderson (2009). "A simple two-stage model predicts response time distributions." *Journal of Physiology* **587**: 4051–4062.

Carpenter, R. H. S. and J. G. Robson, eds. (1998). *Vision Research: A Practical Guide to Laboratory Methods.* Oxford, Oxford University Press.

Carpenter, R. H. S. and M. L. L. Williams (1995). "Neural computation of log likelihood in the control of saccadic eye movements." *Nature* **377**: 59–62.

Chandna, A., D. P. Chandrasekharan, A. V. Ramesh and R. H. S. Carpenter (2012). "Altered interictal saccadic reaction time in migraine: a cross-sectional study." *Cephalalgia* **32**: 473–480.

Chocholle, R. (1940). "Variation des temps de réactions auditifs en fonction de l'intensité à diverses fréquences." *L'année psychologique* **41**: 65–124.

Christie, L. S. and R. D. Luce (1956). "Decision structure and time relations in simple choice behaviour." *Bulletin of Mathematical Biophysics* **18**: 89–112.

Condy, C., S. Rivaud-Péchoux, F. Ostendorf, C.-J. Ploner and B. Gaymard (2004). "Neural substrate of antisaccades." *Neurology* **63**: 1571–1578.

Cournot, A. (1843). *Exposition de la théorie des chances et des probabilités.* Paris.

Craik, K. J. W. (1952). *The Nature of Explanation.* Cambridge, Cambridge University Press.

Crawford, T. J. (1996). "Transient motion of visual texture delays saccadic eye movements." *Acta Psychologica* **92**: 251–262.

Croone, W. (1667). *De ratione motus musculorum.* Amstelodami, Apud Casparum Commelinum

Crosby, E. C. and J. W. Henderson (1948). "The mammalian midbrain and isthmus regions: II. Fibre connections of the superior colliculus. B. Pathways concerned in automatic eye movements." *Journal of Comparative Neurology* **88**: 53–91.

Cunniffe, N., H. Munby, S. Chan, et al. (2015). "Using saccades to diagnose covert hepatic encephalopathy." *Metabolic Brain Disease* **30**: 821–828.

Cutsuridis, V., V. Kumari and U. Ettinger (2014). "Antisaccade performance in schizophrenia: a neural model of decision making in the superior colliculus." *Frontiers in Neuroscience* **8**: 13.

Cutsuridis, V., N. Smyrnis, I. Evdokimidis and S. Perantonis (2007). "A neural model of decision-making by the superior colicullus in an antisaccade task." *Neural Networks* **20**: 690–704.

Cynader, M. and N. Berman (1972). "Receptive-field organization of monkey superior colliculus." *Journal of Neurophysiology* **35**: 187–201.

da Vinci, L. (1998). Notebook, quoted in Carlo Vecce, *Leonardo*. Rome, Salerno.

Dale, A. (1991). *A History of Inverse Probability*. New York, Springer.

Dawson, C., E. Murphy, C. Maritz, et al. (2011). "Dietary treatment of phenylketonuria: the effect of phenylalanine on reaction time." *Journal of Inherited Metabolic Disease* **34**: 419–454.

de Finetti, B. (1937). "La prévision: ses lois logiques, ses sources subjectives." *Annales de l'Institut Henri Poincaré* **7**: 1.

Dempster, A. P. (1968). "A generalization of Bayesian inference." *Journal of the Royal Statistical Society Series B* **30**: 205–247.

Deneve, S. (2008). "Bayesian spiking neurons I: inference." *Neural Computation* **20**: 91–117.

Deneve, S. (2008). "Bayesian spiking neurons II: learning." *Neural Computation* **20**: 118–145.

Descartes, R. (1656). *Discours de la méthode.* Leiden.

Dodge, R. (1900). "Visual perception during eye movement." *Psychological Review* **7**: 454–465.

Dodge, R. (1905). "The illusion of clear vision during eye movement." *Psychological Bulletin* **2**: 193–199.

Dodge, R. and T. S. Cline (1901). "The angle velocity of eye movements." *Psychological Review* **8**: 145–157.

Dolmenech, P. and J.-C. Dreher (2010). "Decision threshold modulation in the human brain." *Journal of Neuroscience* **30**: 14305–14317.

Dryden, J. (1687). *The Hind and the Panther: A Poem, in Three Parts*. London, Jacob Tonson.

Edwards, A. W. F. (1972). *Likelihood.* Cambridge, Cambridge University Press.

Edwards, A. W. F. (1974). "The history of likelihood." *International Statistics Review* **42**: 9–15.

Edwards, A. W. F. (1992). *Likelihood.* Cambridge, Cambridge University Press.

Edwards, A. W. F. (2000). "Fisher information and the fundamental theorem of natural selection." *Istituto Lombardo Rendiconti Scienze* **B134**: 3–17.

Ejima, Y. and Y. Ohtani (1987). "Simple reaction time to sinusoidal grating and perceptual integration time: contributions of perceptual and response processes." *Vision Research* **27**: 269–276.

Emeric, E. E., J. W. Brown, L. Boucher, et al. (2007). "Influence of history on saccade countermanding performance by humans and macaque monkeys." *Vision Research* **47**: 35–49.

Epelboim, J., J. R. Booth and R. M. Steinman (1994). "Reading unspaced text: implications for theories of reading eye movements." *Vision Research* **34**: 1735–1766.

Evarts, E. V., M. Kimura, R. H. Wurtz and O. Hikosaka (1984). "Behavioural correlates of activity in basal ganglia neurons." *Trends in Neuroscience* **77**: 449–453.

Everitt, B. J. and T. W. Robbins (1997). "Central cholinergic systems and cognition." *Annual Review of Psychology* **48**: 649–684.

Evinger, C. and A. F. Fuchs (1978). "Saccadic, smooth pursuit and optokinetic eye movements of the trained cat." *Journal of Physiology* **285**: 209–229.

Fatt, P. and B. Katz (1950). "Some observations on biological noise." *Nature* **166**: 597–598.

Fechner, G. T. (1860). *Elemente der Psychophysik*. Leipzig, Breithopf and Härtel.

Fecteau, J. H. and D. P. Munoz (2003). "Exploring the consequences of the previous trial." *Nature Reviews in Neuroscience* **4**: 1–9.

Fecteau, J. H. and D. P. Munoz (2007). "Warning signals influence motor processing." *Journal of Neurophysiology* **97**: 1600–1609.

Ferraina, S., M. Paré and R. H. Wurtz (2002). "Comparison of cortico-cortico and cortico-collicular signals for generation of saccadic eye movements." *Journal of Neurophysiology* **87**: 845–858.

Ferrier, D. (1886). *The Functions of the Brain.* 2nd ed. London, Smith Elder: xxiii + 498.

Fischer, B. and R. Boch (1983). "Saccadic eye movements after extremely short reaction times in the monkey." *Brain Research* **260**: 21–26.

Fischer, B. and R. Boch (1984). Express saccades of the monkey: a new type of visually guided rapid eye movement after extremely short reaction times. *Theoretical and Applied Aspects of Eye Movement Research.* A. G. Gale and F. Johnston, eds. Amsterdam, Elsevier: 403–408.

Fischer, B., S. Geleck and W. Huber (1995). "The three-loop model: a neural network for the generation of saccadic reaction times." *Biological Cybernetics* **72**: 185–196.

Fischer, B. and J. Krüger (1974). "The shift-effect in the cat's lateral geniculate nucleus." *Experimental Brain Research* **21**: 225–227.

Fischer, B. and E. Ramsperger (1984). "Human express saccades: extremely short reaction times of goal directed eye movements." *Experimental Brain Research* **57**: 191–195.

Fischer, B. and H. Weber (1993). "Express saccades and visual attention." *Behaviour and Brain Research* **16**: 553–610.

Fischer, B., H. Weber, M. Biscaldi, et al. (1993). "Separate populations of visually guided saccades in humans: reaction times and amplitudes." *Experimental Brain Research* **92**: 528–541.

Fisher, R. A. (1921). "On the 'Probable Error' of a coefficient of correlation." *Metron* **1** (Part 4): 3–32.

Fisher, R. A. (1934). "Indeterminism and natural selection." *Philosophy of Science* **1**: 99–117.

Fisher, R. A. (1934). "Randomisation, and an old enigma of card play." *Mathematical Gazette* **18**: 294–297.

Fisher, R. A. (1935). "The logic of inductive inference." *Journal of the Royal Statistical Society* **98**: 39–54.

Fisher, R. A. (1950). *Creative Aspects of Natural Law.* Cambridge, Cambridge University Press.

Flourens, J. (1911). *Encyclopædia Britannica.* 11th ed. Cambridge, Cambridge University Press.

Fuchs, A. F. (1967). "Saccadic and smooth pursuit eye movements in the monkey." *Journal of Physiology* **191**: 609–631.

Furneaux, S. and M. F. Land (1999). "The effects of skill on the eye-hand span during musical sight reading." *Proceedings of the Royal Society B* **266**: 1435–1440.

Gauss, C. F. (1809). *Theoria motvs corporvm coelestivm in sectionibvs conicis Solem ambientivm.* Hamburg, Friderich Perthes.

Genest, W., R. Hammond and R. H. S. Carpenter (2016). "The random dot tachistogram: a novel task that elucidates the functional architecture of decision." *Nature Scientific Reports* **6**: 30787.

Ghosh, B. C. P., R. H. S. Carpenter and J. B. Rowe (2013). "A longitudinal study of motor, oculomotor and cognitive function in progressive supranuclear palsy." *PLoS ONE* **8**.

Gilden, D. L., T. Thornton and M. W. Mallon (1995). "1/f noise in human cognition." *Science* **267**: 1837–1839.

Glimcher, P. W. (2008). The neurobiology of individual decision making, dualism, and legal accountability. *Better than Conscious?* C. Engel and W. Singer, eds. Cambridge, MA, MIT Press: 319–346.

Glimcher, P. W. and A. Rusticini (2004). "Neuroeconomics: the consilience of brain and decision." *Science* **306**: 447–451.

Goard, M. and Y. Dan (2009). "Basal forebrain activation enhances cortical coding of natural scenes." *Nature Neuroscience* **12**: 1444–1449.

Gold, J. I. and M. N. Shadlen (2007). "The neural basis of decision-making." *Annual Review of Neuroscience* **30**: 525–574.

Good, I. J. (1950). *Probability and the Weighing of Evidence*. London, Griffin.

Good, I. J. (1952). "Rational decisions." *Journal of the Royal Statistical Society Series B* **14**: 107–114.

Good, I. J. (1955). "Some terminology and notation in information theory." *Proceedings of the Institute of Electrical Engineers C* **103**: 200–204.

Good, I. J. (1959). "Kinds of probability." *Science* **129**: 443–447.

Good, I. J. (1968). "Corroboration, explanation, evolving probability, simplicity and a sharpened razor." *British Journal of the Philosophy of Science* **19**: 123–143.

Good, I. J. (1971). The probabilistic explication of information, evidence, surprise, causality, explanation and utility. *Foundations of Statistical Inference*. V. P. Godambc and D. A. Sprott, eds, Toronto, Holt, Rinehart and Winston: 108–141.

Good, I. J. (1975). "Explicativity, corroboration and the relative odds of hypotheses." *Synthese* **30**: 39–73.

Gottlieb, J. and M. E. Goldberg (1999). "Activity of neurons in the lateral interparietal area of the monkey during an antisaccade task." *Nature Neuroscience* **2**: 906–912.

Gould, P. and R. White (1974). *Mental Maps*. Harmondsworth, Penguin.

Green, D. M. and R. D. Luce (1971). "Detection of auditory signals presented at random." *Perception and Psychophysics* **9**: 257–268.

Green, D. M. and J. A. Swets (1966). *Signal Detection Theory and Psychophysics*. New York, Wiley.

Gregory, R. L. (1956). An experimental treatment of vision as an information source and noisy channel. *Information Theory*. C. Cherry, ed. London, Butterworth: 287–299.

Grice, G. R. (1968). "Stimulus intensity and response evocation." *Psychological Review* **75**: 359–373.

Grice, G. R., R. Nullmeyer and V. A. Spiker (1977). "Application of variable criterion theory to choice reaction time." *Perception and Psychophysics* **22**: 431–449.

Hacking, I. (1965). *Logic of Statistical Inference*. Cambridge, Cambridge University Press.

Hacking, I. (1975). *The Emergence of Probability*. Cambridge, Cambridge University Press.

Hallett, P. E. and B. D. Adams (1980). "The predictability of saccadic latency in a novel voluntary oculomotor task." *Vision Research* **20**: 329–339.

Halliday, J. and R. H. S. Carpenter (2010). "The effect of cognitive distraction on saccadic latency." *Perception* **39**: 41–50.

Handford, M. (1987). *Where's Wally*. London, Walker.

Hanes, D. P. and R. H. S. Carpenter (1999). "Countermanding saccades in humans." *Vision Research* **39**: 2777–2791.

Hanes, D. P. and J. D. Schall (1995). "Countermanding saccades in macaque." *Visual Neuroscience* **12**: 929–937.

Hanes, D. P. and J. D. Schall (1996). "Neural control of voluntary movement initiation." *Science* **274**: 427–430.

Hänzi, S., H. Copley and R. H. S. Carpenter (2011). "Saccadic latency and information foraging." *Journal of Physiology Proceedings* **23**: PC299.

Harris, C. (1989). "The ethology of saccades: a non-cognitive model." *Biological Cybernetics* **60**: 401–410.

Hebb, D. O. (1949). *Organization of Behaviour*. London, Wiley.

Helmholtz, H. v. (1867). *Handbuch der physiologischen Optik*. Hamburg, Voss.

Henmon, V. A. C. and F. L. Wells (1914). "Concerning individual differences in reaction times." *Psychological Review* **27**: 153–156.

Hershey, L. A., L. Whicker, L. A. Abel, et al. (1983). "Saccadic latency measurements in dementia." *Archives of Neurology* **40**: 592–593.

Hick, W. E. (1952). "On the rate of gain of information." *Quarterly Journal of Experimental Psychology* **4**: 11–26.

Hikosaka, O., Y. Takikawa and R. Kawagoe (2000). "Role of the basal ganglia in the control of purposive saccadic eye movements." *Psychological Review* **80**: 953–978.

Hikosaka, O. and R. H. Wurtz (1983a). "Visual and oculomotor functions of monkey substantia nigra pars reticulata. I. Relation of visual and auditory responses to saccades." *Journal of Neurophysiology* **49**: 1230–1253.

Hikosaka, O. and R. H. Wurtz (1983b). "Visual and oculomotor functions of monkey substantia nigra pars reticulata. II. Visual responses related to fixation of gaze." *Journal of Neurophysiology* **49**: 1254–1267.

Hikosaka, O. and R. H. Wurtz (1983c). "Visual and oculomotor functions of monkey substantia nigra pars reticulata III. Memory-contingent visual and saccadic responses." *Journal of Neurophysiology* **49**: 1268–1284.

Hikosaka, O. and R. H. Wurtz (1983d). "Visual and oculomotor functions of monkey substantia nigra pars reticulata. IV. Relation of substantia nigra to superior colliculus." *Journal of Neurophysiology* **49**: 1285–1301.

Hildreth, J. D. (1973). "Bloch's Law and a temporal integration model." *Perception and Psychophysics* **14**: 421–432.

Hohle, R. H. (1965). "Inferred components of reaction times as functions of foreperiod duration." *Journal of Experimental Psychology* **69**: 382–386.

Holmes, G. (1936). "Looking and seeing." *Irish Journal of Medical Science* **11**: 565–576.

Howie, D. (2002). *Interpreting Probability*. Cambridge, Cambridge University Press.

Hughlings Jackson, J. (1884). "On the evolution and the dissolution of the nervous system." *British Medical Journal* **1 (1213)**: 591–593.

Hughlings Jackson, J. (1932). *Selected Writings*. London, Hodder and Stoughton.

Hume, D. (1739). *A Treatise of Human Nature*. London, Noon.

Hutton, S. B. and U. Ettinger (2006). "The antisaccade task as a research tool in psychopathology: a critical review." *Psychophysiology* **43**: 302–313.

Hutton, S. B., E. M. Joyce, T. R. Barnes and C. Kennard (2002). "Saccadic distractibility in first-episode schizophrenia." *Neuropsychologia* **40**: 1729–1736.

Hyman, R. (1953). "Stimulus information as a determinant of reaction time." *Journal of Experimental Psychology* **45**: 188–196.

James, W. (1890). *Principles of Psychology*. New York, Henry Holt.

Javal, E. (1879). "Essai sur la physiologie de la lecture." *Annales d'oculometrie* **82**: 242–253.

Jeffrey, R. (1965). *The Logic of Decision*. New York, McGraw-Hill.

Jeffreys, H. (1931). *Scientific Inference*. Cambridge, Cambridge University Press.

Jeffreys, H. (1936). "Further significance tests." *Proceedings of the Cambridge Philosophical Society* **32**: 416–445.

Jeffreys, H. (1939). *Theory of Probability*. Oxford, Clarendon Press.

Jenkins, T. N. (1926). "Facilitation and inhibition." *Archives of Psychology* **14**(86): 1–56.

Johnson, H. M. (1918). "The influence of the distribution of brightness over the visual field on the time required for discriminative responses to visual stimuli." *Psychobiology* **1**: 459–494.

Joyce, J. (1922). *Ulysses*. Paris, Shakespeare and Co.

Just, M. A. and P. A. Carpenter (1980). "A theory of reading: from eye fixations to comprehension." *Psychological Review* **87**: 329–354.

Kaas, J., ed. (2009). *Evolutionary Neuroscience*. Oxford, Academic Press.

Kalesnykas, R. P. and P. E. Hallett (1987). "The differentiation of visually guided and anticipatory saccades in gap and overlap paradigms." *Experimental Brain Research* **68**: 115–121.

Kendall, M. G. (1961). *A Course in the Geometry of n Dimensions*. London, Griffin.

Kendall, M. G. and A. Stuart (1968). *The Advanced Theory of Statistics*. London, Griffin.

Keynes, J. M. (1921). *A Treatise on Probability.* London, Macmillan.

Khan, O., S. J. Taylor, J. G. Jones, et al. (1999). "Effects of low-dose isoflurane on saccade eye movement generation." *Anaesthesia* **54**: 142–145.

Khoo, M. C. K. (2000). *Physiological Control Systems: Analysis: Simulation and Estimation.* New York, IEEE Press.

Kiani, R. and M. N. Shadlen (2009). "Representation of confidence associated with a decision by neurons in the parietal cortex." *Science* **324**: 759–763.

Kiesow, F. (1904). "Über die einfachen Reaktionszeiten der taktilen Belastungsempfindung." *Zeitschrift für Psychologie* **35**: 8–49.

Kintsch, W. (1963). "A response time model for choice behaviour." *Psychometrika* **28**: 27–32.

Kolmogorov, A. (1941). "Confidence limits for an unknown distribution function." *Annals of Mathematical Statistics* **23**: 525–540.

Kornhuber, H. H. and L. Deecke (1965). "Hirnpotentialänderungen beim Willkürbewegungen und passiven Bewegungen des Menschen: Bereitschaftspotential und reafferente Potentiale." *Pflügers Archiv* **284**: 1–17.

Krauzlis, R. and N. Dill (2002). "Neural correlates of target choice for pursuit and saccades in the primate superior colliculus." *Neuron* **35**(2): 355–363.

Krismer, F., J. C. P. Roos, M. Schranz, et al. (2010). "Saccadic latency in hepatic encephalopathy: a pilot study." *Metabolic Brain Disease* **25**: 285–295.

Kubie, L. S. (1954). Psychiatric and psychoanalytic considerations of the problem of consciousness. *Brain Mechanisms and Consciousness.* E. D. Adrian, F. Bretler, H. H. Jasper and J. F. Delafresnaye, eds. Oxford, Blackwell: 444–469.

La Berge, D. L. (1962). "A recruitment theory of simple behaviour." *Psychometrika* **27**: 375–396.

La Berge, D. L. and J. R. Tweedy (1964). "Presentation probability and choice time." *Journal of Experimental Psychology* **68**: 477–481.

Laming, D. (1968). *Information Theory of Choice Reaction Times.* New York, Academic.

Laming, D. (1973). *Mathematical Psychology.* London, Academic.

Land, M. F. (1995). The functions of eye movements in animals remote from man. *Eye Movement Research: Mechanisms, Processes and Applications.* J. M. Findlay, R. Walker, R. W. Kentridge, eds. Amsterdam, Elsevier: 63–76.

Land, M. F. and P. McLeod (2000). "From eye movements to actions: how batsmen hit the ball." *Nature Neuroscience* **3**: 1340–1345.

Land, M. F., N. Mennie and J. Rusted (1999). "The roles of vision and eye movements in the control of activities of daily living." *Perception* **28**: 1311–1328.

Land, M. F. and B. W. Tatler (2009). *Looking and Acting.* Oxford, Oxford University Press.

Laplace, P. S. (1812). *Théorie analytique des probabilités.* Paris, Courcier.

Latimer, K. W., J. L. Yates, M. L. Meister, A. C. Huk and J. W. Pillow (2015). "NEURONAL MODELING. Single-trial spike trains in parietal cortex reveal discrete steps during decision-making." *Science* **349** (6244): 184–187.

Laurentius (A du Laurens), A. (1599). *A Discourse of the Preservation of the Sight: of Melancholike Diseases; of Rheumes and of Old Age.* London, Ralph Jackson.

Lauwereyns, J. (2010). *The Anatomy of Bias: How Neural Circuits Weigh the Options.* Cambridge, MA, MIT Press.

Lauwereyns, J., Y. Takikawa, R. Kawagoe, et al. (2002). "Feature-based anticipation of cues that predict reward in monkey caudate nucleus." *Neuron* **33**: 316–318.

Lauwereyns, J., K. Watanabe, B. Loe and O. Hikosaka (2002). "A neural correlate of response bias in monkey caudate nucleus." *Nature* **418**: 413–417.

Lazebnik, Y. (2002). "Can a biologist fix a radio? – Or, what I learned while studying apoptosis." *Cancer Cell* **2**: 179–181.

Leach, J. C. D. and R. H. S. Carpenter (2001). "Saccadic choice with asynchronous targets: evidence for independent randomisation." *Vision Research* **41**: 3437–3445.

Lee, C. S. and R. D. Luce (1956). "Decision structure and time relations in simple choice behaviour." *Bulletin of Mathematical Biophysics* **18**: 89–112.

Lee, D. (2008). "Game theory and neural basis of social decision making." *Nature Neuroscience* **11**: 404–409.

Leigh, R. J. and C. Kennard (2004). "Using saccades as a research tool in the clinical neurosciences." *Brain* **127**: 460–477.

Leigh, R. J. and D. S. Zee (2015). *The Neurology of Eye Movements*. New York, Oxford University Press.

Lenoir, M., L. Crevits, M. Goethals, et al. (2000a). "Saccadic eye movements and finger reaction times of table tennis players of different levels." *Neuro-ophthalmology* **24**: 335–338.

Lenoir, M., L. Crevits, M. Goethals, J. Wildenbeest and E. Musch (2000b). "Are better eye movements an advantage in ball games? A study of prosaccadic and antisaccadic eye movements." *Perceptual and Motor Skills* **91**: 546–552.

Leth-Steensen, C., Z. K. Elbaz and V. I. Douglas (2000). "Mean response times, variability, and skew in the responding of ADHD children: a response time distributional approach." *Acta Psychologica* **104**: 167–190.

Libet, B., D. K. Peall, D. E. Morledge, et al. (1991). "Control of the transition from sensory detection to sensory awareness in man by the duration of a thalamic stimulus." *Brain* **114**: 1731–1757.

Libet, B., E. W. Wright, B. Feinstein and D. K. Pearl (1979). "Subjective referral of the timing for a conscious sensory experience. A functional role for the somatosensory specific projection system in man." *Brain* **102**: 193–224.

Libet, J. (1985). "Subjective antedating of a sensory experience and mind-brain theories: reply to Honderich (1984)." *Journal of Theoretical Biology* **114**: 563.

Lindley, D. V. (1956). "On a measure of the information provided by an experiment." *Annals of Mathematical Statistics* **27**: 986–1005.

Lindley, D. V. (2000). "The philosophy of statistics." *The Statistician* **49**: 293–337.

Llinas, R. (1974). "Motor aspects of cerebellar control." *The Physiologist* **17**: 19–46.

Logan, G. D. and W. B. Cowan (1984). "On the ability to inhibit thoughts and action: a theory of an act of control." *Psychological Review* **91**: 295–327.

Lucas, J. R. (1970). *The Concept of Probability*. Oxford, Clarendon.

Luce, R. D. (1959). *Individual Choice Behaviour: A Theoretical Analysis*. New York, Wiley.

Luce, R. D. (1960). Response latencies and probabilities. *Mathematical Models in the Social Sciences*. K. J. Arrow, S. Karlin and P. Suppes, eds. Stanford, CA, Stanford University Press: 298–311.

Luce, R. D. (1986). *Response Times: Their Role in Inferring Elementary Mental Organization*. London, Oxford University Press.

Ludwig, C. J. H., I. D. Gilchrist and E. McSorley (2005). "The remote distractor effect in saccade programming: channel interaction and lateral inhibition." *Vision Research* **45**: 1177–1190.

Lynch, J. C., V. B. Mountcastle, W. H. Talbot and T. C. T. Yin (1977). "Parietal lobe mechanism for directed visual attention." *Journal of Neurophysiology* **40**: 362–389.

Mach, E. (1875). *Grundlinien der Lehre von den Bewegungsempfindungen*. Leipzig, W Engelmann.

Mach, E. (1886). *Beiträge zur Analyse der Empfindungen*. Jena, Fischer.

Mackay, M., M. Cerf and C. Koch (2012). "Evidence for two distinct mechanisms directing gaze in visual scenes." *Journal of Vision* **12**: 1–12.

Makert, A. and M. Flechtner (1989). "Saccadic reaction times in acute and remitted schizophrenia." *European Archives of*

Psychiatry and Neurological Science **239**: 33–38.

Maxwell, J. C. and W. D. Nivin, eds. (1890). *The Scientific Papers of James Clerk Maxwell.* New York, Dover.

May, R. M. (1976). "Simple mathematical models with very complicated dynamics." *Nature* **261**: 459–467.

McDonald, S. A., R. H. S. Carpenter and R. C. Shillcock (2005). "An anatomically-constrained, stochastic model of eye movement control in reading." *Psychological Review* **112**: 814–840.

McDowell, J., M. Myles-Worsley, H. Coon, W. Byerley and B. Clementz (1999). "Measuring liability for schizophrenia using optimized antisaccade stimulus parameters." *Psychophysiology* **36**: 138–141.

McGill, W. J. (1963). Stochastic latency mechanisms. *Handbook of Mathematical Psychology.* R. D. Luce, R. R. Bush and E. Galanter, eds. London, John Wiley: 309–360.

McGill, W. J. and J. Gibbon (1965). "The general gamma distribution and reaction time." *Journal of Mathematical Psychology* **2**: 1–18.

McIlwain, J. T. (1966). "Some evidence concerning the physiological basis of the periphery effect in the cat's retina." *Experimental Brain Research* **1**: 265–271.

Merleau-Ponty, M. (1945). *Phénomènolgie de la perception.* Paris, Gallimard.

Merrison, A. F. A. and R. H. S. Carpenter (1994). "Co-variability of smooth and saccadic latencies in oculomotor pursuit." *Ophthalmic Research* **26**: 158–162.

Merrison, A. F. A. and R. H. S. Carpenter (1995). "'Express' smooth pursuit." *Vision Research* **35**: 1459–1462.

Meyniel, C., S. Rivaud-Péchoux, P. Damier and B. Gaymard (2005). "Saccade impairments in patients with fronto-temporal dementia." *Journal of Neurology, Neurosurgery and Psychiatry* **76**: 1581–1584.

Michell, A. W., Z. Xu, D. Fritz, et al. (2006). "Saccadic latency distributions in Parkinson's disease and the effects of

L-dopa." *Experimental Brain Research* **169**: 237–245.

Micko, H. C. (1969). "A psychological scale for reaction time measurement." *Acta Psychologica* **30**: 324–335.

Milstein, D. M. and M. C. Dorris (2007). "The influence of expected value on saccadic preparation." *Journal of Neuroscience* **27**: 4810–4818.

Missal, M. and E. L. Keller (2002). "Common inhibitory mechanism for saccades and smooth-pursuit eye movements." *Journal of Neurophysiology* **88**: 1880–1892.

Mollon, J. D. and M. R. Baker, eds. (1995). *The Use of CRT Displays in Research on Colour Vision.* Colour Vision Deficiencies.

Mollon, J. D. and A. J. Perkins (1996). "Errors of judgment at Greenwich in 1796." *Nature* **380**: 101–102.

Munoz, D. P., L. T. Armstrong, K. A. Hampton and K. D. Moore (2003). "Altered control of visual fixation and saccadic eye movements in attention-deficit hyperactivity disorder." *Journal of Neurophysiology* **90**: 503–514.

Munoz, D. P., J. R. Broughton, J. E. Goldring and I. T. Armstrong (1998). "Age-related performance of human subjects on saccadic eye movement tasks." *Experimental Brain Research* **121**: 391–400.

Munoz, D. P. and P. S. Istvan (1998). "Lateral inhibitory interactions in the intermediate layers of the monkey superior colliculus." *Journal of Neurophysiology* **79**: 1193–1209.

Munoz, D. P. and R. H. Wurtz (1993a). "Fixation cells in monkey superior colliculus. 1. Characteristics of cell discharge." *Journal of Neurophysiology* **70**: 559–575.

Munoz, D. P. and R. H. Wurtz (1993b). "Fixation cells in monkey superior colliculus. 2. Reversible activation and deactivation." *Journal of Neurophysiology* **70**: 576–589.

Munoz, D. P. and R. H. Wurtz (1993c). "Superior colliculus and visual fixation." *Biomedical Research* **14**: 75–79.

Munoz, D. P. and R. H. Wurtz (1995). "Saccade-related activity in monkey superior colliculus. I. Characteristics of burst and build-up cells." *Journal of Neurophysiology* **73**: 2313–2333.

Nachev, P., C. Kennard and M. Husain (2008). "Functional role of the supplementary and pre-supplementary motor areas." *Nature Reviews in Neuroscience* **9**: 856–869.

Nagel, E. (1936). "The meaning of probability." *Journal of the American Statistical Association* **31**: 10–30.

Nakahara, H., K. Nakamura and O. Hikosaka (2006). "Extended LATER model can account for trial-by-trial variability of both pre- and post-processes." *Neural Networks* **19**: 1027–1046.

Nettelbeck, T. (1980). Factors affecting reaction time: mental retardation, brain damage, and other psychopathologies. *Reaction Times*. A. T. Welford, ed. New York, Academic Press: 355–401.

Nieuwenhuys, R. (1985). *Chemoarchitecture of the Brain*. Berlin, Springer Verlag.

Noda, H., R. Asoh and M. Shibaki (1977). Floccular unit activity associated with eye movements and fixation. *The Control of Gaze by Brainstem Neurons*. R. Baker and A. Berthoz, eds. New York, Elsevier: 371–380.

Noorani, I. (2014). "LATER models of neural decision behavior in choice tasks." *Frontiers in Integrative Neuroscience* **8**: 67.

Noorani, I. (2017). "Towards a unifying mechanism for cancelling movements." *Philosophical Transactions of the Royal Society B: Biological Sciences* **372**(1718).

Noorani, I. and R. H. Carpenter (2014). "Basal ganglia: racing to say no." *Trends in Neurosciences* **37**(9): 467–469.

Noorani, I. and R. H. Carpenter (2014). "Re-starting a neural race: anti-saccade correction." *European Journal of Neuroscience* **39**(1): 159–164.

Noorani, I. and R. H. Carpenter (2017). "Not moving: the fundamental but neglected motor function." *Philosophical Transactions of the Royal Society B: Biological Sciences* **372**(1718): 20160190.

Noorani, I. and R. H. S. Carpenter (2011). "Full reaction time distributions reveal the complexity of neural decision-making." *European Journal of Neuroscience* **33**: 1948–1951.

Noorani, I. and R. H. S. Carpenter (2013). "Antisaccades as decisions: LATER model predicts latency distributions and error responses." *European Journal of Neuroscience* **37**: 330–338.

Noorani, I. and R. H. S. Carpenter (2015). "Ultra-fast initiation of a neural race by impending errors." *Journal of Physiology* **593**: 4471–4484.

Noorani, I. and R. H. S. Carpenter (2016). "The LATER model of reaction time and decision." *Neuroscience & Biobehavioral Reviews* **64**: 229–251.

Noorani, I., M. J. Gao, B. C. Pearson and R. H. Carpenter (2011). "Predicting the timing of wrong decisions with LATER." *Experimental Brain Research* **209**(4): 587–598.

Nouraei, S. A. R., N. de Pennington, J. G. Jones and R. H. S. Carpenter (2003). "Dose-related effect of sevoflurane sedation on the higher control of eye movements and decision-making." *British Journal of Anaesthesia* **91**: 175–183.

Nouraei, S. A. R., J. C. P. Roos, S. R. Walsh, et al. (2010). "Objective assessment of the hemisphere-specific neurological outcome of carotid endarterectomy: a quantitative saccadometric analysis." *Neurosurgery* **67**: 1534–1541.

Ober, J. K., E. Przedpelska-Ober, W. Gryncewicz, et al. (2003). Hand-held system for ambulatory measurement of saccadic durations of neurological patients. *Modelling and Measurement in Medicine*. J. Gajda, ed. Warsaw, Komitet Biocybernityki i Inzyneierii Biomedycznej PAN: 187–198.

O'Regan, J. K. (1984). How the eye scans isolated words. *Theoretical and Applied Aspects of Eye Movement Research*. A. G. Gale and F. Johnston, eds. Amsterdam, Elsevier: 159–168.

Oswal, A., M. Ogden and R. H. S. Carpenter (2007). "The time-course of stimulus expectation in a saccadic decision task." *Journal of Neurophysiology* **97**: 2722–2730.

Otto, T. U. and P. Mamassian (2012). "Noise and correlations in parallel perceptual decision making." *Current Biology* **22**: 1–6.

Ozyurt, J., H. Colonius and P. Arndt (2003). "Countermanding saccades: evidence against independent processing of go and stop signals." *Perception and Psychophysics* **65**: 420–428.

Pacut, A. (1977). "Some properties of threshold models of reaction latency." *Biological Cybernetics* **28**: 63–72.

Pacut, A. (1980). "Mathematical modelling of reaction latency: the structure of the models and its motivation." *Acta Neurobiologiae Experimentalis* **40**: 199–215.

Patterson, W. F. and J. D. Schall (1997). "Supplementary eye field studied with the countermanding paradigm." *Society for Neuroscience Abstracts* **23**: 474.

Pavlov, I. (1927). *Conditioned Reflexes: An Investigation of the Physiological Activity of the Cerebral Cortex*. London, Oxford University Press.

Pearson, B. C., K. R. Armitage, C. W. M. Horner and R. H. S. Carpenter (2007). "Saccadometry: the possible application of latency distribution measurement for monitoring concussion." *British Journal of Sports Medicine* **41**: 610–612.

Peirce, C. S. (1878). "The probability of induction." *Popular Science Monthly*.

Peirce, C. S. (1923). *Chance, Love and Logic*. New York, Harcourt, Brace.

Peitsch, A., A. Hoffman, I. Armstrong, G. Pari and D. P. Munoz (2008). "Saccadic impairments in Huntington's disease." *Experimental Brain Research* **186**: 457–469.

Perneczky, R., B. C. Ghosh, L. Hughes, et al. (2011). "Saccadic latency in Parkinson's disease correlates with executive function and brain atrophy, but not motor severity." *Neurobiology of Disease* **43**: 79–85.

Pike, R. (1973). "Response latency models for signal detection." *Psychological Review* **80**: 53–68.

Pirenne, M. H. (1950). "Descartes and the body-mind problem in physiology." *The British Journal for the Philosophy of Science* **1**: 43–59.

Pirozzolo, F. J. and E. C. Hansch (1981). "Oculomotor reaction time in dementia reflects degree of cerebral dysfunction." *Science* **214**: 349–351.

Platt, M. L. and S. A. Huettel (2008). "Risky business: the neuroeconomics of decision making under uncertainty." *Nature Neuroscience* **11**: 398.

Poincaré, H. (1908). *Science et méthode*. Paris, E. Flammarion.

Poisson, S. D. (1837). *Recherches sur la probabilité des jugements*. Paris, Bachelier.

Popper, K. R. (1959). *The Logic of Scientific Discovery*. London, Hutchinson.

Porterfield, W. (1737). "An essay concerning the motions of our eyes." *Edinburgh Medical Essays and Observations*, **3**: 160–263.

Putukian, M., R. J. Echemendia and S. Mackin (2000). "The acute neuropsychological effects of heading in soccer: a pilot study." *Clinical Journal of Sports Medicine* **10**: 104–109.

Rashbass, C. (1961). "The relationship between saccadic and smooth tracking eye movements." *Journal of Physiology* **159**: 326–338.

Ratcliff, R. (1978). "A theory of memory retrieval." *Psychological Review* **85**: 59–108.

Ratcliff, R., R. H. S. Carpenter and B. A. J. Reddi (2001). "Putting noise into neurophysiological models of simple decision making." *Nature Neuroscience* **4**: 336–337.

Ratcliff, R., T. van Zandt and G. McKoon (1999). "Connectionist and diffusion models of reaction time." *Psychological Review* **106**: 261–300.

Rayner, K. and M. H. Fischer (1996). "Mindless reading revisited: eye movements during reading and scanning are different." *Perception and Psychophysics* **58**: 734–747.

Rayner, K. and A. Pollatsek (1989). *The Psychology of Reading*. Englewood Cliffs, Prentice-Hall.

Rayner, K. and A. Pollatsek (2012). *The Psychology of Reading*. 2nd ed. Englewood Cliffs, Prentice-Hall.

Reddi, B. and R. H. S. Carpenter (2000). "The influence of urgency on decision time." *Nature Neuroscience* 3: 827–831.

Reddi, B. A. J. (2001). "Decision making: the two stages of neuronal judgement." *Current Biology* 11: 603–606.

Reddi, B. A. J., K. N. Asrress and R. H. S. Carpenter (2003). "Accuracy, information and response time in a saccadic decision task." *Journal of Neurophysiology* 90: 3538–3546.

Restle, F. (1961). *Psychology of Judgement and Choice*. New York, Wiley.

Reuter, B. and N. Kathmann (2004). "Using saccade tasks as a tool to analyze executive dysfunctions in schizophrenia." *Acta Psychologica* 115: 255–269.

Reynolds, A. M. (2007). "Free-flight odour tracking in *Drosophila* is consistent with an optimal scale-free search." *PLoS ONE* 2: 4.

Robbins, T. W. (1997). "Arousal systems and attentional processes." *Biological Psychology* 45: 57–71.

Robbins, T. W. (2000). "Chemical neuromodulation of frontal executive functions in humans and other animals." *Experimental Brain Research* 133: 130–138.

Robbins, T. W., S. Granon, J. L. Muir, et al. (1998). "Neural systems underlying arousal and attention." *Annals of the New York Academy of Sciences* 846: 222–237.

Robert, M. P., P. C. Nachev, S. L. Hicks, et al. (2009). "Saccadometry of conditional rules in presymptomatic Huntington's Disease." *Annals of the New York Academy of Sciences* 1164: 444–450.

Robinson, D. A. (1972). "Eye movements evoked by collicular stimulation in the alert monkey." *Vision Research* 12: 1795–1808.

Robinson, D. A. (1981). "The use of control systems analysis in the neurophysiology of eye movements." *Annual Review of Neuroscience* 4: 463–503.

Robinson, D. A., J. L. Gordon and S. E. Gordon (1986). "A model of the smooth pursuit eye movement system." *Biological Cybernetics* 55: 43–57.

Roltman, J. D. and M. N. Shadlen (2002). "Response of neurons in the lateral intraparietal area during a combined visual discrimination reaction time task." *Journal of Neuroscience* 22: 9475–9489.

Roos, J., R. Lachmann, T. Cox and R. Carpenter (2006). "Saccadometry for estimating cerebral damage in storage diseases." *Acta Paediatrica* 95: 141.

Roos, J. C. P., D. M. Calandrini and R. H. S. Carpenter (2005). "The relation between evoked and spontaneous saccadic latencies." *Annals of Neurology* 58.

Roos, J. C. P., D. M. Calandrini and R. H. S. Carpenter (2008). "A single mechanism for the timing of spontaneous and evoked saccades." *Experimental Brain Research* 187: 283–293.

Salinas, E. and T. R. Stanford (2013). "The countermanding task revisited: fast stimulus detection is a key determinant of psychophysical performance." *Journal of Neuroscience* 33: 5668–5685.

Sarnat, H. B. and M. G. Netsky (1974). *Evolution of the Nervous System*. Oxford, Oxford University Press.

Saville, D. J. and G. R. Wood (1996). *Statistical Methods: A Geometric Primer*. New York, Springer.

Schall, J. D. (2000). "Decision making: from sensory evidence to a motor command." *Current Biology* 10: 404–406.

Schall, J. D. (2003). "On building a bridge between brain and behavior." *Annual Review of Psychology* 55: 02.01–02.28.

Schall, J. D. (2004). "On the role of the frontal eye fields in guiding attention and saccades." *Vision Research* 44: 1453–1467.

Schall, J. D. (2005). "Decision making." *Current Biology* 15: R9–R11.

Schall, J. D. and N. Bichot (1998). "Neural correlates of visual and motor processes." *Current Opinion in Neurobiology* 8: 211–217.

Schall, J. D. and D. P. Hanes (1993). "Neural basis of saccade target selection in frontal eye field during visual search." *Nature* 366: 467–469.

Schall, J. D., D. P. Hanes, K. G. Thompson and D. J. King (1995). "Saccade target selection in frontal eye field of Macaque. I. Visual and premovement activation." *Journal of Neuroscience* **15**: 6905–6918.

Schall, J. D., T. J. Palmieri and G. D. Logan (2017). "Models of inhibitory control." *Philosophical Transactions B of the Royal Society: Biological Sciences* **372**(1718): 20160193.

Schall, J. D., V. Stuphorn and J. W. Brown (2002). "Monitoring and control of action by the frontal lobes." *Neuron* **36**: 309–322.

Schall, J. D. and K. G. Thompson (1999). "Neural selection and control of visually guided eye movements." *Annual Review of Neuroscience* **22**: 241–259.

Schiller, P. H. and F. Koerner (1971). "Discharge characteristics of single units in the superior colliculus of the alert Rhesus monkey." *Journal of Neurophysiology* **34**: 920–936.

Schiller, P. H. and M. Stryker (1972). "Single-unit recording and stimulation in superior colliculus of the alert Rhesus monkey." *Journal of Neurophysiology* **35**: 915–924.

Schilling, W. (1921). "The effect of caffein and acetanilid on simple reaction time." *Psychological Review* **28**(1), 72–79.

Schmidt, R., D. K. Leventhal, N. Mallet, F. Chen and J. D. Berke (2013). "Canceling actions involves a race between basal ganglia pathways." *Nature Neuroscience* **16**: 1118–1124.

Schmied, A., M. Benita, H. Conde and J. F. Dormont (1979). "Activity of ventrolateral thalamic neurons in relation to a simple reaction time task in the cat." *Experimental Brain Research* **36**: 285–300.

Schultz, W. (2000). "Multiple reward signals in the brain." *Nature Reviews in Neuroscience* **1**: 199–207.

Schultz, W. (2007). "Multiple dopamine functions at different time courses." *Annual Review of Neuroscience* **30**: 259–288.

Schultz, W. (2016). "Dopamine reward prediction error coding." *Dialogues in Clinical Neuroscience* **18**: 23–32.

Schultz, W. and R. Romo (1992). "Role of primate basal ganglia in the internal generation of movements. I. Preparatory activity in the anterior striatum " *Experimental Brain Research* **91**: 363–384.

Schupp, W. and C. Schlier (1972). "The dependence of simple reaction time on temporal patterns of stimuli." *Kybernetik* **11**: 105–111.

Shadlen, M. N. and J. I. Gold (2004). The neurophysiology of decision-making as a window on cognition. *The Cognitive Neurosciences*. M. S. Gazzaniga, ed. Cambridge, MA, MIT Press: 1229–1241.

Shadlen, M. N. and W. T. Newsome (1996). "Motion perception: seeing and deciding." *Proceedings of the National Academy of Sciences* **93**: 628–633.

Shafer, G. (1991). "Can the various meanings of probability be reconciled?" *University of Kansas, School of Business Working Paper* **230**.

Shakespeare, W. (1595). *A Midsummer Night's Dream*. London, Thomas Fisher.

Shannon, C. E. and W. Weaver (1949). *The Mathematical Theory of Communication*. Urbana, University of Illinois Press.

Shelton, L., L. Beccerra and D. Borsook (2012). "Unmasking the mysteries of the habenula in pain and analgesia." *Progress in Neurobiology* **96**: 208–219.

Sherrington, C. S. (1940). *Man on his Nature*. Cambridge, Cambridge University Press.

Simpson, J. and E. Weiner (1989). *The Oxford English Dictionary*. Oxford, Clarendon Press.

Sinha, N., J. T. G. Brown and R. H. S. Carpenter (2006). "Task switching as a two-stage decision process." *Journal of Neurophysiology* **95**: 3146–3153.

Smart, J. J. C. (955). "Metaphysics, logic and theology." *New Essays in Philosophical Theology*. A. Flew and A. MacIntyre, eds. London, SCM Press: 42–60.

Smirnov, N. V. (1948). "Table for estimating the goodness of fit of empirical distributions." *Annals of Mathematics and Statistics* **19**: 279–281.

Smith, G. A. (1980). Models of choice reaction time. *Reaction Times*. A. T. Welford, ed. New York, Academic Press: 173–214.

Smith, J. E., C. A. Zahn and E. P. Cook (2001). "The functional link between Area MT neural fluctuations and detection of a brief motion stimulus." *Journal of Neuroscience* **31**: 13458–13468.

Smith, K., J. Dickhaut, K. McCabe and J. V. Pardo (2002). "Neural substrates for choice under ambiguity, risk, gains and losses." *Management Science* **48**: 711–718.

Smyrnis, N. (2008). "Metric issues in the study of eye movements in psychiatry." *Brain and Cognition* **68**: 341–358.

Smythies, J. (2009). "Philosophy, perception and neuroscience." *Philosophy* **38**: 638–651.

Sommerville, D. M. Y. (1958). *An Introduction to the Geometry of N Dimensions.* New York, Dover.

Spinoza, B. D. (1993). *Ethics.* London, Everyman.Originally published 1677.

St-Cyr, G. J. (1973). "Signal and noise in the human oculomotor system." *Vision Research* **13**: 1979–1991.

Stam, C. J. (2005). "Nonlinear dynamical analysis of EEG and MEG: review of an emerging field." *Clinical Neurophysiology* **116**: 2266–2301.

Stark, L. (1968). *Neurological Control Systems.* New York, Plenum.

Stone, M. (1960). "Models for choice reaction time." *Psychometrika* **25**: 251–260.

Story, G. W. and R. H. S. Carpenter (2009). "Dual LATER-unit model predicts saccadic reaction time distributions in gap, step and appearance tasks." *Experimental Brain Research* **193**: 287–296.

Stoyan, D., W. S. Kendall and J. Mecke (1995). *Stochastic Geometry and Its Applications.* New York, Wiley.

Tatler, B. W., J. R. Brockmole and R. H. S. Carpenter (2017). "LATEST: a model of saccadic decisions in space and time." *Psychological Review* **124**: 267–300.

Tatler, B. W. and S. B. Hutton (2006). "Trial by trials effects in the antisaccade task." *Experimental Brain Research* **179**(3): 387–396.

Taylor, M. J., R. H. Carpenter and A. J. Anderson (2006). "A noisy transform predicts saccadic and manual reaction times to changes in contrast." *Journal of Physiology* **573**(Pt 3): 741–751.

Temel, Y., V. Visser-Vandewalle and R. H. S. Carpenter (2008). "Saccadic latency during electrical stimulation of the human subthalamic nucleus." *Current Biology* **18**: R412–414.

Thakkar, K., J. D. Schall, G. D. Logan and S. Park (2015). "Response inhibition and response monitoring in a saccadic double-step task in schizophrenia." *Brain and Cognition* **95**: 90–98.

Thier, P. and U. J. Ilg (2005). "The neural basis of smooth-pursuit eye movements." *Current Opinion in Neurobiology* **15**: 645–652.

Thompson, K. G., N. P. Bichot and J. D. Schall (1997). "Dissociation of visual discrimination from saccade programming in macaque frontal eye field." *Journal of Neurophysiology* **77**: 1046–1959.

Thompson, K. G., D. P. Hanes, N. P. Bichot and J. D. Schall (1996). "Perceptual and motor processing stages identified in the activity of macaque frontal eye field neurons during visual search." *Journal of Neurophysiology* **76**: 4040–4055.

Thomson, W. (1884). "Electrical units of measurement." *Popular Lectures and Addresses* I: 73.

Thorpe, S., D. Fize and C. Marlot (1996). "Speed of processing in the human visual system." *Nature* **381**: 520–552.

Tolhurst, D. J. (1975). "Reaction times in the detection of gratings by human observers: a probabilistic mechanism." *Vision Research* **15**: 1143–1149.

Tolstoy, L. (1869). *War and Peace.* The Russian Messenger.

Tyrrell, G. N. M. (1946). *The Personality of Man.* London, Penguin.

Usher, M., J. D. Cohen, D. Servan-Schreiber, J. Rajkowski and G. Aston-Jones (1999). "The role of locus coeruleus in the regulation of cognitive performance." *Science* **283**: 549–554.

van Biervliet, J. (1899). "Noyau d'origine du nerf oculo-moteur commun du lapin." *La cellule* **16**: 1–33.

van den Berg, A. V. and E. M. van Loon (2005). "An invariant for timing of saccades during visual search." *Vision Research* **45**: 1543–1555.

van Hemmen, L. J. (2009). "Editorial to volume 100 of Biological Cybernetics." *Biological Cybernetics* **100**: 1–3.

Van Loon, E., I. T. Hooge and A. Van den Berg (2002). "The timing of sequences of saccades in visual search." *Proceedings of the Royal Society B* **269**: 1571–1579.

Venn, J. (1876). *The Logic of Chance*. London, Macmillan.

Vickers, D. (1979). *Decision Processes in Visual Perception*. New York, Academic.

Vickers, D. (1980). Discrimination. *Reaction Times*. A. T. Welford, ed. New York, Academic: 25–72.

von Neumann, J. and O. Morgenstern (1947). *Theory of Games and Economic Behaviour*. Princeton, Princeton University Press.

Wagenmakers, E.-J., S. Farrell and R. Ratcliff (2004). "Estimation and interpretation of 1/f noise in human cognition." *Psychonomic Bulletin and Review* **11**: 579–615.

Wald, A. (1947). *Sequential Analysis*. New York, Wiley.

Wald, A. and J. Wolfowitz (1948). "Optimum character of the sequential probability test." *Annals of Mathematics and Statistics* **19**: 326–339.

Walls, G. L. (1962). "The evolutionary history of eye movements." *Vision Research* **2**: 69–80.

Walsh, E. G. (1952). "Visual reaction time and the alpha-rhythm, an investigation of the scanning hypothesis." *Journal of Physiology* **118**: 500–508.

Walsh, S. R., S. A. R. Nouraei, T. Y. Tang, et al. (2010). "Remote ischemic preconditioning for cerebral and cardiac protection during carotid endarterectomy: results from a pilot randomized clinical trial." *Vascular and Endovascular Surgery* **44**: 434–439.

Walton, M. M. and N. J. Gandhi (2006). "Behavioral evaluation of movement cancellation." *Journal of Neurophysiology* **96**: 2011–2024.

Ware, J. S., P. R. Blount and R. H. S. Carpenter (2001). The Dynamics of Expectation: Rapid Effects of Probabilistic Cues on Saccadic Latency. Neural Control of Movement: 11th Annual Meeting, Seville.

Watson, A. B. (1979). "Probability summation over time." *Vision Research* **19**: 515–522.

Weatherford, R. (1982). *Philosophical Foundations of Probability Theory*. London, Routledge and Kegan Paul.

Weaver, W. (1948). "Probability, rarity, interest and surprise." *Scientific Monthly* **67**: 390–392.

Weiss, Y. and E. H. Adelson (1998). "Slow and smooth: a Bayesian theory for the combination of local motion signals in human vision." *MIT AI Laboratories Memo* AI Memo 1624.

Welford, A. T. (1959). "Evidence of a single-channel decision mechanism limiting performance in a serial reaction task." *Quarterly Journal of Experimental Psychology* **11**: 193–208.

Welford, A. T., ed. (1980). *Reaction Times*. London, Academic Press.

Wells, G. R. (1913). "Influence of stimulus duration on reaction-time." *Psychological Review Monographs* **15**(5): 1–69.

Wheeless, L. L., R. M. Boynton and G. H. Cohen (1966). "Eye-movement responses to step and pulse-step stimuli." *Journal of the Optical Society of America* **56**: 956–960.

Wheeless, L. L., G. H. Cohen and R. M. Boynton (1967). "Luminance as a parameter of the eye-movement control system." *Journal of the Optical Society of America* **57**: 394–400.

White, C. T., R. G. Eason and N. R. Bartlett (1962). "Latency and duration of eye movements in the horizontal plane." *Journal of the Optical Society of America* **52**: 210–213.

Wickens, T. D. (1995). *The Geometry of Multivariate Statistics*. Mahwah, Lawrence Erlbaum.

Wiener, S. I., C. A. Paul and H. Eichenbaum (1989). "Spatial and behavioural correlates of hippocampal neuronal activity." *Journal of Neuroscience* **9**: 2737–2763.

Wilde, O. (1894). "Phrases and philosophies for the use of the young." *The Chameleon.* Oxford, Oxford University Press.

Wittmann, B. C., N. D. Daw, B. Seymour and R. J. Dolan (2008). "Striatal activity underlies novelty-based choice in humans." *Neuron* **58**: 967–973.

Wolf, C. (1865). "Recherches sur l'équation personelle dans les observations de passages, sa détermination absolue, ses lois et son origine." *Annales de l'Observatoire de Paris: Mémoires* **8**: 153.

Wundt, W. (1862). *Beiträge zur Theorie der Sinneswahrnehmungen.* Leipzig.

Wundt, W. (1887). *Physiologischen Psychologie.* Leipzig.

Wurtz, R. H. and J. E. Albano (1980). "Visual-motor function of the primate superior colliculus." *Annual Review of Neuroscience* **3**: 189–226.

Wurtz, R. H. and M. E. Goldberg (1972). "Activity of superior colliculus in behaving monkey: III. Cells discharging before eye movements." *Journal of Neurophysiology* **35**: 575–586.

Wurtz, R. H. and M. E. Goldberg, eds. (1989). *The Neurobiology of Saccadic Eye Movements.* Amsterdam, Elsevier.

Yang, T. and M. N. Shadlen (2007). "Probabilistic reasoning by neurons." *Nature* **447**: 1075–1080.

Yarbus, A. L. (1967). *Eye Movements and Vision.* New York, Plenum.

Yerkes, R. M. (1903). "A study of the reactions and reaction times of the Medusa Gonionema Murbachii to photic stimuli." *American Journal of Physiology* **9**: 279–307.

Yerkes, R. M. (1904). "Variability of reaction-time." *Psychological Bulletin* **1**: 137–146.

Yoshimatsu, H. and M. Yamada (1991). "High dimensional chaos of miniature eye movements." *Proceedings of the Annual International Conference of the IEEE Engineering in Medicine and Biology Society* **13**: 1513–1515.

Yu, A. J. and P. Dayan (2005). "Uncertainty, neuromodulation, and attention." *Neuron* **46**: 681–692.

Index